'Dilys Daws has inspired generations of parents, children, and fellow professionals. This beautiful collection of her writings reflects the enormous range of her work as a child psychotherapist, trainer, campaigner, and passionate supporter of primary care. She writes with clarity and simplicity. This book will continue to inspire many more people in the future.'

— **John Launer,** *GP; honorary consultant, Tavistock Clinic;*
honorary associate professor, UCL; former
associate dean at Health Education England

'In this collection of papers for the World Series, we finally have a fitting tribute to Daws' contribution to our field, and one that does justice to the breadth and scope of her work. Over the course of her career, Daws has changed the landscape both within child psychotherapy and without. She has fostered change within important allied professions and then worked collaboratively with those allies in psychiatry, health visiting and general medicine through clinical work, campaigning and lobbying. All this and her courage, compassion, curiosity and humour are evident in this important volume.'

— **Dr. Alexandra de Rementeria,** *Editor in Chief of*
the Journal of Child Psychotherapy; Lead Therapist
with the Tavistock Outreach in Primary
Schools project; M7 Assessment Tutor

'Based on over 50 years' observations "standing next to the weighing scales" and Dilys' deep respect for health visitors, this immense collection is a must-read for everyone working with families who are experiencing difficulties. "Quietly Subversive" reminds us to look beyond targets and tasks – families' lives are changed when they feel seen, understood, and supported.'

— **Alison Morton,** *Executive Director,*
Institute of Health Visiting

Quietly Subversive

This book gathers together selected papers and book chapters by Dilys Daws, covering her 50 years of pioneering work as a child psychotherapist.

It provides those working with parents, infants, and children with a means of learning from Daws's decades of experience as a psychotherapist and therapeutic consultant, with plentiful case material illustrating her method of working in action. The first two sections of the book focus on her work as a consultant psychotherapist in the baby clinic of a GP practice and her parent-infant work in this context as well as at the Tavistock and Portman Clinic. The third section explores her work with young children, focusing on questions around the therapeutic frame and setting. The fourth section features extended excerpts from her writings for the general public, most particularly aimed at new parents and parents with infants. Finally, the book also contains several short reflective pieces addressing themes to do with parent-infant work, the experience of the therapist, and the social role of psychoanalytic thinking.

This book will be of interest to all those working with parents and children, including doctors, health visitors, and social workers, as well as child psychotherapists and child psychoanalysts.

Dilys Daws was Consultant Child Psychotherapist at the Tavistock and Portman NHS Foundation Trust where she was awarded a Doctorate and a visiting consultant at the baby clinic of the James Wigg Practice, Kentish Town. She was Chair of the Association of Child Psychotherapists, and Founder Chair of the Association for Infant Mental Health-UK. She has had 50 years of clinical and teaching experience, has lectured on child psychotherapy and infant mental health widely in the UK and abroad, and has politically lobbied for it.

Matthew Lumley has studied at the Tavistock and Portman, where he completed his Post-Graduate Diploma in Working with Children, Young People and Families: A Psychoanalytic Observational Approach. He has worked for many years with autistic children in both primary and secondary school settings, and for two years as an assistant psychotherapist in the Tavistock Outreach in Primary Schools programme.

The World Library of Mental Health

The *World Library of Mental Health* celebrates the important contributions to mental health made by leading experts in their individual fields. Each author has compiled a career-long collection of what they consider to be their finest pieces: extracts from books, journals, articles, major theoretical and practical contributions, and salient research findings.

For the first time ever the work of each contributor is presented in a single volume so readers can follow the themes and progress of their work and identify the contributions made to, and the development of, the fields themselves.

Each book in the series features a specially written introduction by the contributor giving an overview of their career, contextualizing their selection within the development of the field, and showing how their own thinking developed over time.

Recent titles in this series:

Living Archetypes
The Selected Works of Anthony Stevens
Anthony Stevens

Soul: Treatment and Recovery
The Selected Works of Murray Stein
Murray Stein

Existential Psychotherapy and Counselling after Postmodernism
The selected works of Del Loewenthal
Del Loewenthal

Love the Wild Swan
The Selected Works of Judith Edwards
Judith Edwards

For more information about this series, please visit: www.routledge.com

Quietly Subversive
The Selected Works of Dilys Daws

Dilys Daws With Matthew Lumley

Routledge
Taylor & Francis Group

NEW YORK AND LONDON

Cover image: Dilys Daws

First published 2023
by Routledge
605 Third Avenue, New York, NY 10158

and by Routledge
4 Park Square, Milton Park, Abingdon, Oxon, OX14 4RN

Routledge is an imprint of the Taylor & Francis Group, an informa business

Library of Congress Cataloging-in-Publication Data
A catalog record for this book has been requested

ISBN: 978-1-032-29463-6 (hbk)
ISBN: 978-1-032-35030-1 (pbk)
ISBN: 978-1-003-32493-5 (ebk)

DOI: 10.4324/b23125

Typeset in Times New Roman
by Apex CoVantage, LLC

The quiet subversiveness of psychoanalytic thinking! So are subversive and creative the same thing? Subversive means positively turning things over, uprooting. The more negative undermining is only one facet of its meaning.

Contents

Foreword

Dilys Daws has been standing next to the weighing scales in the GP baby clinic for almost half a century. I have never seen her there but can imagine her attentive expression and comforting stillness as she 'eavesdrops on the progress of every baby who attends the clinic.' In an elegant distillation of her history and passions here is Dilys, born in Huddersfield of Russian Jewish ancestry, who studied social anthropology at Cambridge, followed by psychoanalytical child psychotherapy at the Tavistock Clinic, an outsider who is also an insider.

Her clinical opportunism is more than anthropological participant observation; it is an engagement in the life of a general practice. In the classic 1985 paper with which this book begins, Dilys writes, '[T]he most crucial issue is where to put oneself.' Having found the right spot – the equivalent of the water cooler in an office – she learned how to wait; 'it takes as much skill to stand next to a weighing machine as it does not to talk during a psychotherapy session.' This is psychoanalysis too, an alert curiosity about relatedness that makes a difference to all those present. Like the nativity scene, the infant is centre stage, with a mother and health visitor in attendance. And with their highly evolved vigilance for what is happening between the people around them, babies can be helpful co-therapists (Fivaz-Despeursinge et al, 2010). Sometimes, a brief engagement is enough; remember Donald Winnicott's dictum, '[I]n child psychiatry the motto often must be "How little need I do to make a bridge between conscious and unconscious?"' (Winnicott, 1965).

From this regular presence in primary care came a deepening respect for health visiting, a clinical profession that does not require you to have a problem. As her father, Jack Kahn, was a GP until he joined the new NHS (in which he became a distinguished child psychiatrist) Dilys was already impressed by what family doctors could do. Live consultations in the baby clinic became a crucible of learning and change for all the participants (*Enlivened or Burnt Out*) but also lit a spark of near-evangelism for a greater understanding of these nicely timed opportunities – like a surfer catching a wave – that can alter the trajectory of a family's life. Dilys's initiative in supporting the creation of the Institute of Health Visiting raised the profile of this often-threatened and misunderstood gem of British public health, while her foundation in 1996 of the UK Association for Infant Mental Health has been a triumph, affecting not only great numbers of early years professionals but also national policy.

Though I have not found the word anywhere in this book, Dilys is a *systemic* psychoanalytical therapist. While child psychotherapy is inevitably a family intervention, we read here also of strategic contacts with others involved in the child's life, in primary care, education, and social services. Besides the baby clinic, here is another example. School refusal is one of the most intractable problems in child mental health practice. On the anniversary of his father's death, 11-year-old Leo was in a psychosomatic panic about school and would not go. Dilys thought that having therapy would ease the boy's sorrow but might not loosen the special bond with his widowed mother. So she offered him two sessions a week *on condition* that he first returned to school. Though 'horrified by my obtuseness and hardness' (*p. 109 in the original 1986 'Consent' paper*) and awed by the containing coalition between therapist, mother, and social worker, Leo returned to school and made good use of therapy during the following year.

Quietly Subversive is a clever title, because Dilys does not appear to be making a noise, yet she has with some cunning and great deal of determination shifted the consciousness of generations of people who work with and care for children, which of course includes parents. There is spirited playfulness here, but it is really serious, and learned. Meeting Dilys at the weighing scale, you would not know of her scholarship but will find yourself the focus of unhurried interest in whatever it is you have to tell her.

Sebastian Kraemer

References

Fivaz-Despeursinge, E., Lavanchy-Scaiola, C., & Favez, N. (2010). 'The young infant's triangular communication in the family: Access to threesome intersubjectivity? Conceptual considerations and case illustrations'. *Psychoanalytic Dialogues*, 20 (2): 125–40.

Winnicott, D. W. (1965). 'Child therapy: A case of anti-social behaviour: "Mark" aet 12 years'. In: J. G. Howells (Ed.), *Modern Perspectives in Child Psychiatry*. London: Oliver & Boyd, pp. 523–33. [reprinted in Winnicott's *Collected Works*, 2017, p. 525.10:3:15]

Memoir

I was born in Huddersfield in the West Riding of Yorkshire to a Russian-Jewish family. My father was a GP, working from home, and my mother helped him run it. Today, she would be the practice manager. The house they had built just before I was born was exciting, a flat-roofed Bauhaus design, unique among the usual traditional Yorkshire stone-built houses, and maybe a symbol of my father's progressive ideas. Perhaps being brought up in it helped lead me towards my own 'quietly subversive' ideas! After the war, my father trained as a child psychiatrist. I was 13 then, old enough to be fascinated by what he was reading and talking about. There was Freud on the dining-room table! I was also influenced by my mother's 'style', her love of babies, her ability to listen, and her creativity with the family and home. She also later trained as a Marriage Guidance Counsellor. I was inspired by the excitement of their work and thought I also wanted to be a doctor.

Near the end of secondary school, I realised I was good at the arts but not at science. I could learn science but not think about it and be creative. Instead of medicine I did Social Anthropology at Newnham College, Cambridge, and loved doing it. Meyer Fortes was the Professor, and Edmund Leach the Reader. They were psychoanalytically minded so it was a really good start. After my degree, I did a year as a research assistant to Meyer Fortes and then moved to London and was a research assistant at the Institute of Community Studies with Michael Young and other inventive minds of the late 1950s, looking at how people live, their interrelations and their social context. I piloted a study for Ann Cartwright about patients' experience in hospital and found that even using a questionnaire I got a real conversation going, and at the end people would say 'Thank you. I feel much better.' That is when I discovered that talking was a helpful kind of therapy!

I then had the grandiose idea to connect psychoanalysis and social anthropology and spoke to various people about it. Elizabeth Spillius (who had done both) was encouraging, but when I got to see the social scientist Marie Jahoda, she gave me the most sensible advice: 'Go and do one of them properly.'

My father then gave me useful advice to become a child psychotherapist and in fact having done social anthropology gave me a wider view to it. I did the training at the Tavistock Clinic, splendidly run by Mattie Harris. I was interviewed by Dr Bowlby, who in suggesting an analyst said, 'Why don't you go to a friend of mine, Pearl King?' She was an Independent analyst, then called 'Middle Group,' and a really good choice for me, though the training was largely Kleinian. She was a wise, slightly rebellious person, part of the establishment but also critical of it, so a bit like me, or I'm a bit like her!

I trained with Juliet Hopkins, also an Independent, and we've been friends and worked together ever since. We have been in a peer supervision group with Eileen Orford and recently the essential younger colleague Janine Sternberg who is always there to give me advice! Very differently to now, the training was only three years in length, including the infant observation with Mrs. Bick, and we both stayed on for another year because three years was not enough, continuing with our training cases and our analyses, and went to many lectures again.

We both got married about then. My first husband Lawrence Daws was an Australian painter and we spent a year travelling, with time in Australia, where I worked in a clinic seeing child patients and supervising most of the clinicians. For six months, Adelaide was connected with Kleinian theory! I knew more of it at that moment than ever before or since! On my return, I was pregnant and took five years off from clinical work, although doing some lecturing and writing, as well as being Hon. Sec. of the ACP. My first writing was the book *Your One Year Old*, one of a Tavistock series of mini books about each age of children. I was asked to do it by Dina Rosenbluth who was running out of time for her own deadline. I had only two months to do it in, a week to find a minder for my baby in the mornings while my three-year-old was at nursery, a week to plan what to write, and six weeks to interview friends with one-year-olds and write the short book. I was lucky to have been able to do this with the recent tutors from my training. I am sure it freed me up for confidence in writing various books and papers during my career.

In 1971, I joined the Child Guidance Training Centre (CGTC) and its Day Unit. A publisher friend suggested I write a book comparing Freud and Jung. I knew this was not one of my abilities, but it led me to think of producing the first British book on child psychotherapy. I started editing this, and Mary Boston joined me and we edited *The Child Psychotherapist and Problems of Young People*. The draft began with the word 'Although' and the Wildwood publisher Dieter Pevsner said, 'You'll never change the world with although!' The best interpretation I have ever had.

Dieter obviously realised that I wanted to change the world! My being 'quietly subversive' is about that. Subversive means positively turning things over, uprooting. The more negative meaning of undermining is only one facet of its meaning. One of the first changes that I created was through my work as a visiting psychotherapist at the baby clinic of the James Wigg practice, which I started in 1975. After having my second baby, I had had some problems and went back to my analyst to discuss my anxieties. She was very helpful, and I wondered, 'Who would I have gone to if I had not been in the therapeutic world?' I thought that there should be someone easily available in primary care and that I should be that person. After a few years at the CGTC and its Day Unit, I talked to the medical director John Bolland and then to Alexis Brook at the Tavistock who introduced me to the James Wigg practice, and I was there for 45 years. My interest in infant mental health started there. I have really enjoyed the clinical work, and the consultations with GPs and Health Visitors. The practice generously told me that I 'changed the way they worked.' Though I believe they already connected body and mind in the way they thought about their patients, and I was deeply impressed with the atmosphere of the Practice. After working with the health visitors, I have described them as being 'the emotional safety-net for parents and babies.' Many of my former trainees now also work in GP practices. Families can much more easily seek brief help within the practice that they feel they belong to.

In 1985, I started my adult psychoanalytic psychotherapy training with the BAP, now the BPF – an extra, enjoyable dimension to my professional life. That same year the CGTC merged with the Tavistock, and I became a consultant child psychotherapist in the Child and Family Department, with my work there also gradually concentrating on infant mental health – co-leading the Under Fives Counselling Service and the Infant Mental Health Workshop with Lisa Miller and Juliet Hopkins, with influence from Mary-Sue Moore visiting from the United States, and helping set up the PGdip/MA in Infant Mental Health with Juliet and Paul Barrows, to be run by Louise Emanuel. In 1989, my book *Through the Night: Helping Parents and Sleepless Infants* came out and was a crucial part of defining my career.

While I was Chair of the Association of Child Psychotherapists, I realised one day that three of us four officers meeting in a room in London were from Yorkshire, including myself. I wondered why we were all there and not still in the North! My own clinical work, teaching, and consultation have led me to want to spread my ideas to other professions especially Health Visitors, and to other parts of the country, as part of the Tavistock's 'mission.' The feeling of security offered to me by being part of the CGTC and then the Tavistock made me able to do this. As Chair of the Child Psychotherapy Trust, I then encouraged those colleagues who were setting up trainings outside London, in alliance with the Tavistock, especially Margaret Rustin. My husband Eric Rayner, an Independent psychoanalyst, whose mother came from Liverpool, similarly helped spread psychoanalysis across the country and we encouraged each other in doing this. The main aim of the CPT was to get child psychotherapy known by the government and the public. I was able to successfully lobby the government, a crucial part of this was getting them to agree to establishing and funding the training of child psychotherapists within the NHS, which was then negotiated by the ACP. I and colleagues were also writing and speaking in the media about child psychotherapy and infant mental health to spread awareness and inform the public.

Belonging to the World Association for Infant Mental Health (WAIMH), I attended and spoke at many of their World Congresses. I also belonged to a European study group meeting in Paris twice yearly, convened by Antoine

Guedeney, and saw how it underpinned the formation of WAIMH-France. In 1995, Eric and I spoke at a regional conference of the Australian AIMH. I was impressed with the way that the various professions involved with infants and their families got together. On the long plane journey home, I thought, 'We could do that!' Inspiration born of boredom! Back home I wrote to several different professionals, all of whom replied positively and we set up AIMH-UK in March 1996. They included Juliet Hopkins, Lynne Murray, Sebastian Kraemer, Penelope Leach, Joan Raphael Leff, and Christine Puckering, all of whom have remained close to it. AIMH-UK has been successful in connecting many professionals and supporting front-line workers with the psychodynamic ideas they have previously missed out on. Jane Barlow, the current President has greatly increased its effect.

It has also had an impact on WAIMH. My closest colleagues there, especially in Congress Symposia, have been Astrid Berg, Antoine Guedeney, Campbell Paul, Frances Thomson Salo, and Stephen Seligman. We have similar aims and inspire each other in spreading the influence of infant mental health round the world.

I have also had much help and companionship in writing books. Recently *Through the Night*, originally published by Robert Young and edited by Ann Scott for FAB, was updated with the help of Sarah Sutton (2021). Later, John Launer, who has taught GPs about psychotherapy and psychotherapists about work in GP practices, edited with Sue Blake and myself *Reflecting on Reality: Psychotherapists at Work in Primary Care* (2005). Wanting to get ideas out to parents, I wrote a book with a younger Tavistock colleague, Alexandra de Rementeria, then on maternity leave. The book *Finding Your Way with Your Baby: The Emotional Life of Parents and Babies* (2015) won the BMA Medical Books Awards 1st prize for Popular Medicine in 2016 (updated 2021).

Much of my work has been in disseminating psychoanalytic ideas and in supporting front-line workers in other professions, in both writing and teaching around the country and abroad, and in political lobbying. Being 'quietly subversive' is about doing just that, helping to change ideas in a way that is manageable and makes people feel better about themselves.

Dilys Daws

Introduction

This book gathers together in one place a selection of papers that represent the full breadth of Dilys Daws's extensive and varied contributions to the field of child psychotherapy during her 50 years as a practitioner. Indeed, the sheer range of uses that she has found for the role of psychotherapist is perhaps one of the defining features of her career – working as a consultant in the public services and as a parent-infant and child psychotherapist in an array of different settings, writing uniquely psychoanalytically informed baby books for parents, lobbying government to advocate for psychotherapeutic approaches to mental health as chair of the Child Psychotherapy Trust, and founding AIMH-UK. For this reason, rather than being arranged chronologically, the papers have been selected and grouped in such a way as to reflect these diverse facets of her work, as well as to highlight the unifying through-lines, with their shared roots in a deep commitment to the social value of psychoanalysis.

The first two parts focus on the two distinct but closely interrelated main aspects of her work as a psychotherapist in the baby clinic of a GP practice. Part 1 addresses her role as a psychotherapeutic consultant, working closely with the staff at the practice (primarily doctors and health visitors) to share and spread awareness of psychodynamic ways of thinking about the problems of parents and infants who use the clinic, and to provide therapeutic support to frontline workers. The first paper, 'Standing next to the weighing scales,' is now widely considered a classic and addresses the consultant therapist's literal and symbolic positioning of themselves within the organisation of the clinic, as well as the dynamics involved in the therapist's presence as an 'outsider' and the ways in which they can use their stance to create spaces for reflective thinking among staff-members. The second paper, 'Standing by the weighing scales 30 years on,' returns to these themes, reflecting more broadly on the work done by the clinic and the wide range of ways in which the consultant therapist can enhance and support it. These papers are followed by a reflective piece entitled 'Psychoanalysis and the public service: can they inspire each other?,' which considers more generally the possibility for a mutually beneficial relationship between psychoanalysis and the public services.

The second part addresses her role as a parent-infant psychotherapist within this context, as well as at the Tavistock Clinic, and her work carrying out brief psychoanalytic interventions with parents and infants who might not otherwise have access to this kind of support. Her papers on this area discuss the most common problems that she has seen in her work (namely sleeping and feeding issues, postnatal depression, and mothers' difficulties in bonding with their baby) and her approach based on the thesis that disturbed behaviour in infants is often the result of difficulties arising in the parent or parental couple. 'The baby in the consulting room' contains Dilys's fullest account of her therapeutic technique and discusses the importance of having the baby present in the therapy sessions, as well as the complexities involved in being attuned to a family. 'Brief psychoanalytic therapy for sleep problems' is originally a book chapter and looks in detail at working therapeutically with sleep problems in infants, examining common dynamics within the family that often underlie these problems, suggesting how these can be addressed by brief interventions, and comparing this approach with behavioural schools of thought. 'Feeding problems and relationship difficulties' considers in depth the particularities and differences involved in working with infants who are feeding either too much or too little. The final paper in this part, 'The perils of intimacy' is a ground-breaking study that examines the question of distance and closeness in feeding and weaning and looks at dynamics of separation involved in the weaning process – with particular attention paid to possible psychological meanings of the spoon.

In part 3, the focus turns to Dilys's work with young children in a Day Unit attached to the Child Guidance Training Centre, where she first worked, and later at the Tavistock Clinic. The two papers in this section not only look at the therapeutic process but also importantly examine the framework and the context in which it takes place. The first paper, 'Consent in child psychotherapy' examines the complexities surrounding consent to psychotherapeutic intervention. Much of the significance and originality of this paper lies in its addressing of the often-overlooked question of the child's consent to the therapeutic method and the way in which achieving this consent may form a part of the therapy itself. It also discusses the importance of the therapist's relationship with the parents and argues that work should be done to maintain the parents' consent throughout the duration of the therapy. The second paper in this section, 'Resistance and co-operation: the need for both' looks at Dilys's work as child psychotherapist in a Day Unit. It examines the ambivalent feelings towards therapy and the therapist that are often present within institutions and how this can lead to resistance to the work, as well as suggesting the value of working with this resistance and navigating complex professional boundaries in order to achieve cooperative relationships with other staff members – in this instance, teachers in the school. A unifying theme of these first three parts, and a major through-line in Dilys Daws's thinking, is the attention given to the psychoanalytically informed work that goes on around the clinical work itself: the careful navigation and management of institutional dynamics and professional relationships that is sometimes as crucial to the success of clinical work as the direct psychotherapeutic intervention.

The fourth part features extended excerpts from Dilys's writings for the general public, most particularly aimed at new parents and parents with infants (up to two years old). These works draw from Dilys's experience of working with parents and infants. Alongside the insight into the emotional lives of parents and their babies that they contain, the importance of these writings for this book lies in the example they give of Dilys's work to make complex psychoanalytic theory relatable and understandable to those outside the field – a crucial dimension of her life's work that has also formed a key part of her consultant role in the baby clinic and as a chair of AIMH. The excerpts have been chosen in such a way as to differ thematically from the accounts of parent-infant psychotherapy in the second section and also to draw out the way in which Dilys's approach to writing 'baby books' has striven to help parents engage with the most difficult and sometimes disturbing emotional aspects of infant life and parenting that are so often glossed over but that are so importantly addressed by psychoanalysis.

Finally, part 5 is comprised of five short reflective pieces, most of which Dilys originally presented at WAIMH symposia (ones mainly convened by her) and that touch thought-provokingly on a variety of issues highly relevant to anyone working in this field. 'Enlivened or burnt out' raises questions about the effect of this work on the practitioner and considers both the toll it can take as well as the benefits it can bestow. 'Saying what you mean, or meaning what you say' was written for *The Bulletin* (ACP magazine) and speaks up against a tendency towards self-infantilisation within the profession of child psychotherapy and 'obsequiousness' in writing about other people's writing. 'Working at the edge: the quiet subversiveness of psychoanalytic thinking' suggests the power of psychoanalytic thinking to channel conflict and discord into creative ways of challenging established norms and injustices. 'Error and repair' discusses how getting it wrong may be part of the process of getting it right, and the necessity of continual self-scrutiny in therapeutic work. Lastly, 'Rivalry with fathers' brings attention to the danger of professionals unconsciously entering into competition with the father when working with mothers and babies and highlights the meaningfulness of the father's actual or symbolic presence.

It is our hope that this book will provide all those working with parents and children – including doctors, health visitors, and social workers as well as child psychotherapists and child psychoanalysts – with a means of learning from Dilys Daws's decades of experience.

Matthew Lumley

Acknowledgements

Joanne Forshaw suggested this book at an ideal moment of my retirement and for several years gave very helpful support to me and my co-writers in getting books published. Frances Thomson Salo and Ann Horne at different stages inspired the title *Quietly Subversive*.

Matthew Lumley has expertly edited the book. I joked that I had only written one paper! He read pieces of mine spanning 50 years and found that was partly true! I was often asked to write or give a talk on the same subject. He chose the best papers on each one, cut out the repetitions, and helped shape them into a book. Working with him has been very enjoyable and has meant having the benefits of a clear younger mind. Catherine Alexander has added some finishing touches.

Thanks to all the families who shared their stories with me. My husband Eric, sons Sam and Will and step-children, their partners, my grandchildren and my friends have given me much encouragement with writing. I have mentioned the names of several valued colleagues in my Memoir, and many others were appreciated during my lifetime of work.

Part 1

Therapeutic consultancy

A child psychotherapist in a GP practice

1 Standing next to the weighing scales[1]

Originally published in the Journal of Child Psychotherapy (1985, Vol. 11, No. 2) *and previously given as a paper at a Scientific Meeting of the Association of Child Psychotherapists on 22nd October 1985.*

I have been working for several years in the baby clinic of a general practice in a health centre. One day weekly there are baby clinics, morning and afternoon, each taken by two of the GPs and the four health visitors attached to the practice. A nurse attends to give immunisations. I now go weekly to the morning clinics. I have contact with the other doctors in the practice and at times work closely with the practice's social worker who is a qualified psychotherapist.

I originally started to work at this baby clinic with a thesis that many mothers of new babies may have difficulties arising from their own personalities and from previous relationships, which become reflected in their dealings with the baby, or in disturbed behaviour of some kind in the baby. Mothers who had had no serious difficulties at other periods of their lives might have been thrown off balance by the experience of pregnancy, childbirth, and caring for a very new baby. I hoped that brief psychotherapeutic work of a combined interpretative and supportive nature could relieve some of these problems. Work could be directly with the mother, or mother and father, or by supporting the doctor or health visitor already involved with the family. The majority of babies are routinely brought for clinic visits by their mothers and I believe this influences the nature of my referrals. I see more mothers and babies together than mothers and fathers and babies. Usually, this seems an appropriate way of working; at other times it may be symptomatic of a marital or family problem.[2] In the several years I have worked in the baby clinic, I have felt my ambition to carry out short-term pieces of work has been justified.

The issues that have arisen over these years are of two main kinds. One is the nature of the clinical work undertaken. (Much of this presents as sleep problems, and I give an account of this work in the companion paper which follows.) The second is the process of being a consultant to an institution other

DOI: 10.4324/b23125-2

than one's own. I use the term 'consultant' charily: it is not intended as a confusion with the medical use of the term.

As a 'consultant' from outside, the most crucial issue is where to put oneself. At first, I thought this to be a personal, idiosyncratic problem; it took time to generalise it. An outside professional can be useful in bringing specific skills and knowledge to an institution. Is being an outside consultant or, more baldly, an outsider, of value in itself? Having outsiders around can make a group feel uncomfortable. Being an outsider in such a group is uncomfortable. From our potty training days on, we strive to be acceptable members of a social group. Elenore Smith Bowen has described in 'Return to Laughter' (1954) how lonely and difficult it is to be an anthropologist living in a primitive culture. While one is occupied in questioning the natives on the details of their kinship patterns, all is well. When night draws in and the anthropologist hears laughter from the nearby huts, she feels excluded and wonders if she is the subject of the laughter. It is apparent, however, that her usefulness as an anthropologist remains only if she continues to study kinship – if she settles in to become a part of the culture, her scientific value is endangered.

How does this analogy apply to the child psychotherapist in a baby clinic of a general practice?

When I started work at this practice, Dr. Alexis Brook, who had introduced me to it, offered to support me with monthly discussions on my work there. These were very valuable at first in my newness and tentativeness. Then I began to feel disloyal to the practice, talking about my contacts there 'behind their backs' so to speak. I regret now that I did not voice these feelings to Alexis Brook; I might have learned much sooner what being a 'consultant' is about. As it was, I strove for a feeling of 'belonging' in my once-weekly visits to the practice. In my defence I may say that the atmosphere there is warm and welcoming, appreciated by staff and patients alike.

At this time I sought to do a great deal of clinical work, feeling myself to be a useful member of the primary health care team, seeing the parents and babies thought to be in particular need by their GP or health visitor. Two problems then emerged. The busier I was, the less visible. If I was really energetic and really co-operative, I could see four families, or mothers and babies, in four hours. I would end up bemused by details of feeding and sleeping patterns, or parents' relationships with their own parents, and hopelessly confused. It would be galling to emerge from this to find a health visitor saying, 'I haven't seen you all morning. I didn't know you were here.' It seemed that visibility was an attribute in itself. Secondly, whenever I got a referral, it was rarely soon enough. I would see parents with an eight-month-old baby who had slept badly since birth. They had been patients of the practice for those eight months. I had been visiting for those eight months. Why had I not seen them earlier?

I began to realise that talking about patients was as important as being shut away seeing a few, and that much of my usefulness was in sharing ideas about the problems of mothers and babies with my colleagues, furthermore, that the timing of good referrals was partly dependent on the timing of informal discussions with me. I realised I must be visible, available, and receptive.

I first learnt how to stand next to the weighing scales during vacant hours when a patient had cancelled an appointment. Gradually, I realised it might be the optimal place to be. It is the focal point of the baby clinic: near the reception desk; near the chairs where mothers sit and chat, holding their babies, or watching their small children play on the floor; where the health visitors welcome each mother and assess how much or how little help she is asking for that day; where the doctors come out to greet patients or chase up information.

Bringing the baby to be weighed is the focus for the baby clinic. Parents can visit with no other ostensible reason than to weigh the baby. This alone validates the visit while enabling the mother or father to make use of a contact with the health visitor or make friends with other parents. The moment of weighing the baby can symbolically represent, rationally or not, the total state of development of the baby. A gain of weight can confirm for a mother that her feeding and care have done the baby good; a loss of weight may set the alarm bells going for all concerned. The value of these measurements is not as irrefutable evidence but as an illustration of what sensitive health care workers have already divined as going on between each mother and baby. Standing by the weighing scales is thus an effective way of eavesdropping on the progress of every baby who attends the clinic.

It takes as much skill to stand next to a weighing machine as it does not to talk during a psychotherapy session. My patients sometimes complain of my silence and I think, 'Me, silent? I've been thinking hard all the time.' The skill of thinking on behalf of the patient is only evident if one says in words one's thoughts; if one talks too much, reflective thought has no time to grow.

Standing doing nothing equally requires skill if it is not to be puzzling and persecuting to the people around. It is legitimised in a busy clinic because members of all professions stand at times looking around, sometimes assessing what to do next, sometimes talking to each other. I could be any of these, standing receptively to watch what is going on, or immediately available for discussion. If I am too self-contained, it must seem that my observations are for some unexplained private use; if I am too efficiently outgoing, mothers hand me their baby books to check them into the clinic.

By watching, I gain what for me is invaluable – seeing a whole range of mothers and babies interact. Weekly, my store of impressions of normality and pathology is reinforced so that when someone is referred to me with a problem, I have a background of knowing where this might fit in with what usually happens between mothers and babies, get the chance to talk, informally, at times of less stress, to mothers I have previously worked with, and see how the baby has developed, without further problems needing to be a reason for our meeting. This is a luxury we rarely have in a Child Guidance Clinic.

Most important, by being physically present at the routine baby clinic, I hope to be available for those responsible for the babies to be able to cross-check their own impressions of whether things are going well or badly for a particular baby and its parents. A meeting at the end of the baby clinic briefly reviews each attendance. By having been around, I am a more credible part of this discussion. I do not believe that I am the only holder of a psychodynamic viewpoint. We would do well to acknowledge, as members of the psychotherapy professions, that we came to these professions because psychoanalytic thinking is embedded in present-day culture – the culture did not arise because of us. Our contribution is to keep it in circulation in spite of our own as well as our colleagues' many resistances. In the baby clinic, my colleagues have specific medical and nursing skills; they also have a basic underlying psychodynamic approach to their patients. My task is in reinforcing this approach in my colleagues, not in allowing it to be attributed only to me.

I have described myself as centrally placed in the baby clinic – can I persist in calling myself an outsider? I hope so. I hope I do not stop questioning the shared assumptions of the baby clinic. The very acceptance of many disturbed and disturbing people, something that this practice does so well, in itself creates problems. It can lead to a forgetting that some of their behaviours or their problems might be changed; my role is sometimes to highlight this. An outsider who does not have the responsibility for the management and continuance of the baby clinic can listen out for the reverberances that these patients cause in the workers who try to help them. These reverberances are a useful diagnostic tool if they can be recognised as such.

One problem in this kind of consultative work is in the process of continuity. Because I have visited the practice for a long time, and feel at home there, I expect that the staff know me and are used to working with me. I forget that with each new partner or health visitor, or change-over of trainee doctor, I must do more than get to know them in personal terms. I must also let them know what I feel is my function in the practice.

The need for this often becomes evident the first time they attempt to make a referral to me, and I hedge over taking it. In the discussion over whether I should see a particular patient, each of us is forced to spell out our assumptions of what benefit might or might not accrue to the patient if I saw him or her. Talking about the principle behind a referral goes deeper than simply asking what the problems and background of the patient are. It includes looking at what the present and future relationship of referrer (i.e. doctor or health visitor), patient and psychotherapist will be. Individual work that I do with a patient is a direct extension of work done already by the referrer. A good referral comes usually from someone in whom the patient has already entrusted confidences or who at least has shown a crack in the face of their rejection of help. Work done by me will connect back into the routine contact the mother has with the baby clinic. Some referrals are made from long, close contact with the patient. The referral letters from one woman's senior partner contain as much information and insight about the patient as I am likely to acquire in several weeks of hourly sessions. Where the doctor-patient relationship has achieved so much, the contacts with me may need to be validated for the patient with frequent visits to the GP about physical symptoms. At other times, I suspect that the urgency of patients' demands makes the worker feel that for me to see a patient would rescue both worker and patient alike.

In spite of all my reservations, I do accept many referrals and perhaps have learnt not to disappear from sight while seeing patients. To that end, I always mention the referrer to new patients, with the implication that I will discuss their progress with him or her. In only a few cases has confidentiality that excluded the doctor or health visitor been necessary for confidence to be placed in me.

In the context of a group general practice, doctors and others see themselves as part of a team intervening at different moments over a period of years. Some patients will faithfully attend one doctor, except in emergencies, but often the transference is shared by the practice as a whole, or some members in it, with the actual named doctor of that patient. The transference to me personally has a variety of meanings to different patients. This depends partly on how casually or how formally the referral has been set up. In an atmosphere of informal goodwill, it may seem stuffy to insist on use of surnames, formal referral letters, and deferred appointments, but I believe that a professional distance still has value. I rarely see a patient the same day, even if I happen to be free. When I do, I often feel that there has not been the same therapeutic impact in the consultation as one in which the patient has had time to prepare herself, time to work out the balance of vulnerability and defences, which will enable her to use this session as more than an emergency outpouring of her troubles.

Although my particular interest is in the problems of new babies, children under the school age of five are the province of this clinic. Problems of all this age range of children are discussed with me. I am more chary of taking on children over five. It often makes sense to see parents for a consultation on a puzzling stage of development in their child. Such brief informal work has obvious supportive and informative use and may help prevent problems from increasing. It can, however, leave a child and family with less flexibility in the possibility of other treatment. Granted some families might come once or twice to their own doctor's surgery who would never manage the formality of clinic appointments. Some brief interpretative work might be an opportunity they would never otherwise have. With other cases, I feel that seeing me first complicates an eventual referral. I have neither the brief nor the time to run a miniature child guidance clinic, but I can also see how irritating this position might be to the GPs. Many emotional and behavioural problems of children over five are brought to them in the course of their surgeries. There is not the easy supportive forum of the baby clinic for the doctor to discuss these older children. He can offer either more time at the end of his own surgery or a formal outside referral to a Child Guidance Clinic.

One main issue about a referral is whether it is more helpful for me to see the patient myself or to use the approach from the concerned colleague as a chance to discuss together the problems involved. Often a doctor or health visitor needs simply a fresh view of their patient's problems, not a fresh person to see them.

Next is the issue of whether to take a referral as being meant for oneself, or as an assessment to refer on to another agency, usually of course a Child Guidance Clinic. Referring patients from an institution one is involved in to another such is insurpassable as an opportunity to be seen to be wrong in two places at once. In each situation, the intermediary is seen as an intrinsic member of the other team. By definition, one institution seems to misunderstand how to make a proper referral, and the other to misunderstand what to do with one.

Setting this aside, a too quick assumption that patients should be passed on seems to dismay the referring doctor. One who makes many excellent referrals to me had a couple of recent ones that I had then passed on to our Child Guidance Clinic recommended for intensive therapy. He said he had not thought of them as being so disturbed. One of the strengths of an experienced GP is that he has seen a lot of children grow up and seen families tolerate a lot of disturbed behaviour. It may not be helpful if he feels that I as a psychotherapist panic every time I meet a child showing some disturbance and head them off away from the practice.

Doctors are used to making many referrals of patients. Good doctors are used to discussing the referral with the patients in such a way that the patient feels the referral to be an extension of the doctor's own care, not a rejection of the patient, nor as a giving up in despair by the doctor. What doctors are not so used to doing is discussing a referral at length with the colleague to whom they are making it. I feel that this is one of my main functions in the practice. It is also the hardest to manage and the hardest to explain.

Discussing the case makes obvious sense as an opportunity for me to be given information about the patient, about the problem, and some of the background. All I need to do is ask for more details, enquire why the referral is being made at this particular moment, express my interest, and my intention of keeping the referrer informed. This may be a successful interchange. Some brief psychotherapy has been economically set up, convenient for the patients, and quite often successful enough. Why not settle for as many such cases as I can pick up?

It seems as though struggling with the reason for a referral still makes sense, not only to evaluate whether I could help this particular patient but also in terms of a need to make the work done with the patient as known as possible to the referrer. I can see busy doctors trying to hide their impatience. They are torn daily by their need to deal with medical emergencies and get through a long list of appointments and their awareness that some patients need time to talk about their problems. They have to juggle these two kinds of needs and feel that what I can offer is the luxury of time to a few selected patients. By contrast, I feel that much of my value to the practice is in reporting back my conclusions on how referral symptoms connect with family relationships. It takes time to relate this convincingly and the doctor may think he is not saving much time if he listens to it. I am not the only one who can make such connections – I was only invited to work in this practice because of the awareness already there. But if the doctor does listen to my conclusions, he will be supported in increasingly seeing such connections when families tell him of their problems. Additional insight brings additional responsibilities. The more he recognises problems, the more he will feel the need to listen, and to worry. His work will increase beyond bearing, either in time or accumulated anxiety.

Contained in this is one answer to my earlier question, 'Why do I so often get a referral "too late"?' Perhaps it is impossible for doctors and health visitors to receive the full impact of the pathology of every patient they see. In fact, the baby clinic is a 'well-baby' clinic, and much of the work is in supporting normality and healthy development. In order for such a clinic to survive, there must be a basic assumption that the anxieties brought constantly are being by definition met and dealt with by the routine activities of the clinic.

Mothers, and fathers, particularly with first babies, may have an infinite dread that they are unable and unworthy to look after a baby properly and that the proof of this will be that the baby does not survive. For many of these, the weekly confirmation that their baby has survived, even that it is doing well, becomes a validation for the mother by her health visitor and doctor that she is being a good-enough mother. Something that perhaps was not worked out with the mother's own mother, the permission to be a good mother, becomes worked out through this weekly interchange. The workers in the baby clinic have to stand this projected anxiety weekly and survive for the parents until the next week. Sharing the anxiety can protect the worker; passing it on in the form of a referral can break the experience of the baby clinic as a bulwark of continuing mothering.

Similarly, doctors know that patients use a consultation with them as a focus for cumulative anxiety about their child. How does a doctor distinguish between a consultation where anxiety is communicated and satisfactorily contained for the patient within that consultation, from one where the signal is to use outside help? The feelings stirred up in the doctor do not always help to distinguish. Consultations that leave the doctor feeling anxious and helpless may have been highly successful from the point of view of a patient who goes off relieved of a burden. The doctor's efforts to produce additional help for the patient may mystify someone who already feels much better. Conversely, other patients are unable to say how bad things really are – they protect themselves and workers alike with a facade of well-turned-out babies. Doctors and health visitors have to do sensitive detective work to prise out the agonies of broken nights or other difficulties in relationships between babies and parents.

In a careful baby clinic, the end-of-clinic meeting reviews every attendance, and worries about each baby and family seen are spoken and noted. These meetings inform the workers involved and this information is then an enriched background to every contact each member of the team has with that family. The meeting also enables the workers to share the experience of aroused anxiety that has accumulated during the three hours or more of the baby clinic. It serves as a process of working through that enables the workers to go home no longer invaded by a total experience of anxieties communicated and absorbed, but not openly interpreted as in a psychotherapy session. The positive use to these meetings is thus obvious. Should we, however, worry about whether their use as a resolution of anxiety for the workers mediates against a continuity of action on behalf of the patient?

The converse problem for health-care workers is in the giving up of their omnipotence. Health visitors have an obligation to visit all new babies, and it is rarely that they are refused access to the home for this visit. After this, unless there is grave cause for concern about how a baby is being treated, visits by families to the clinic, or by workers to the home, are conducted on the basis that families are voluntarily using professional services set up for their benefit. Professionals have to wait to be consulted, and they have to think carefully of what they are being asked to do. Like good grandparents, they do not use their own experience to take over parenting from the parents: perhaps they provide a model of availability and receptivity to the parents' anxieties, which enables the parents to do the same for their babies.

What I hope to have done in this paper is to have spelt out the complexity of being a 'consultant,' that is, an outsider in an institution, involved at the point where anxiety can effectively be aroused or allayed. The process of being involved in the referral of patients means being involved with the referrer at a moment of working out which is in the best interests of both patients and the workers.

The unexpressed underlying theme might be what happens to all this anxiety when it touches the consultant weekly. Being an outsider enables the consultant to be free of shared defences and thus free to pick out anxieties. This same outside position means he does not have continued responsibility for the institution and can perhaps leave the anxieties behind on going home. Paradoxically, the most effective resolution for me of the anxieties aroused is in the clinical work I undertake at the baby clinic. Work with albeit a few selected patients can represent a working through of the cumulative mass of problems raised at the clinics.

I believe that I, as an outsider, help my insider colleagues continually to look at the assumptions on which their clinic is run. Perhaps what all such clinics need is not necessarily an outside person, but the flexibility to put themselves from time to time outside their institution in order to question how useful it really is to the patients who come to it.

Acknowledgement

With thanks to the James Wigg Practice at the Kentish Town Health Centre for giving me standing room.

Notes

1 My title echoes Dr. Hyla Holden's phrase 'propping up the filing cabinet,' coined in similar circumstances.
2 Because the majority of patients are women, I shall use 'she' and 'her' to denote them. The majority of doctors in this practice when I started there were men and I shall use 'he' and 'him' to denote them.

Reference

Bowen Smith, E. (1954). *Return to Laughter*. London: Gollancz.

2 A child psychotherapist in the baby clinic of a general practice

Standing by the weighing scales 30 years on

Originally published as a chapter in **Reflecting on Reality: Psychotherapists At Work in Primary Care** *(ed. Launer J., Blake S., and Daws D.) An earlier version was published as a paper in* **Clinical Child Psychology and Psychiatry** *(1999, Vol. 4).*

Just over 30 years ago I started work at the baby clinic of a GP practice: the James Wigg Practice in Kentish Town, London. I called my first paper on work there 'Standing next to the weighing scales' (Daws, 1985). I am gratified that this phrase has caught on with some of my colleagues, and I hear them jokingly say, 'This is standing by the weighing scales kind of work' when they talk about their ventures into various settings. I wrote then about the difficulties of doing this work, and even though the practice I visit is friendly and welcoming, of feeling exposed and vulnerable in an institution not one's own. When asked now about the qualities needed, I usually say: 'a very thick skin'!

Why am I still there 30 years later? As a psychotherapist, I look at patients' present situations in terms of early experience. In the same way, my own interest in working as a child psychotherapist in general practice must have its roots in family experience. My father, Jack Kahn, before training as a psychiatrist, was a GP in Huddersfield in the days when practices were run from the doctor's home. My mother answered the telephone, helped do the accounts, and knew who all the patients were. Today, she would be called the practice manager. As we grew up, my sister and I saw the exhaustion and frustration of this life, but what remains in the memory is the excitement, the essential nature of the work, and the close contacts with the local community. In addition, my father was a town councillor, for some years chairman of the health committee. Huddersfield, in Yorkshire, was a wool-manufacturing town that prided itself on its public health standards; the legend was that Huddersfield was the first to have achieved *general* vaccination in the nineteenth century. Before the NHS, working-men paid a few pence a week to be 'on the panel' and be able to be seen by a GP, but this did not include their wives and children. My father, like many doctors, saw these families for no fee. His income

DOI: 10.4324/b23125-3

came from his (modestly) fee-paying patients. So doctors themselves were running an informal balancing system. This was realistic for those like my father, working in districts where there were also lower-middle- and middle-class patients – not possible in more poverty-stricken areas. So by the time my father left general practice in 1947, I had absorbed the idea that public policies and individual commitment could jointly be powerful forces in preventative health measures.

With the creation of the National Health Service in 1948, the shape of general practice changed greatly. The family doctor charter of 1966 encouraged large group practices; some were set up in specially designed health centres. Multidisciplinary primary care teams developed, including health visitors, practice nurses, and others. Various medical specialists became attached to or visited large general practices. In recent years, this has coincided with a movement from within mental health services to go out into the community.

As the introduction to this book makes clear, the Tavistock Clinic was at the forefront of this development. Following Balint's pioneering work, there was much further study of the essential nature of the therapeutic ingredients of what goes on between doctor and patient, notably by his wife, Enid Balint, and her colleagues (Balint & Norrell, 1973; Balint et al., 1993; M. Balint, 1957). Alexis Brook, who was one of the pioneers in visiting a general practice, trained others, including myself, to help GPs 'increase their skills in identifying and tackling the psychological problems they meet in daily life' (Brook, 1978).

General practitioners have to diagnose, and manage in some way, frankly psychiatric disorders. They also have to deal with the more nebulous connections between physical symptoms and states of mind. Launer (1994) has made a valuable differentiation between the doctor's use of emotional insights in his day-to-day work with patients, leading into 'opportunistic' counselling, contrasting this with formal prearranged counselling either by the GP or by a designated counsellor. He humorously uses the term 'little C' and 'big C' to refer to these. Zalidis (1994), another general practitioner, wrote: 'When a patient feels unwell he or she may present to the general practitioner with symptoms which can be the physical accompaniments of anxiety, or with anxiety that is precipitated by physical symptoms, or a combination of both' (p. 180). The emotional consequences of physical illness and, even more so, the psychic underpinning of many somatic states have been increasingly recognised in general practice. Similarly, Elder (1986) has described the doctor's support at periods when patients are experiencing life events,

> that are some of the psychological determinants of people's lives. . . . Morbidity and presentations to the doctor are known to increase when people are negotiating their major transitions of life, or life events. This means that the doctor is often involved when psychic history is being made. He can, therefore, influence this process a little, for better or for worse.
>
> (p. 75)

A child psychotherapist in the baby clinic

Until recently, counselling and psychotherapy in general practice have mainly been with adults. As in other mental health services, children's needs have been less well recognised. However, the practice in which I work puts children and their families high on the agenda. My connection with the practice is through the baby clinic (Daws, 1995). In the United Kingdom, these clinics are universally available to families with children from birth up to five years. They are staffed by health visitors who are nurses with an additional training and qualification, and also by doctors. The clinics have a statutory function in providing immunisations and routine developmental checks as well as a more informal setting where parents can get advice and support on their infant's progress. In the practice that I visit, two counsellors work with adult patients, and we keep in touch about referrals that might overlap. So I am discussing my consultative role from a personal stance; my colleagues fulfil similar functions.

Since I first visited the practice, I have been going there one morning a week, at a time when a baby clinic is being held. For many young parents, the baby clinic is a crucial institution, for some even a lifeline. The clinic is equally important for the professionals as the focused time of the week in which they see and discuss the infants they are responsible for. By being present during the clinic, I can also, to some extent, be part of its routine and be available to talk about families that doctors and health visitors have on their minds. The development of this work reflects the recent worldwide interest in parent-infant psychotherapy and its applications.

Work in a baby clinic enables families to get help with their infant's development as early as possible; the hope is that later difficulties in the relationship between parents and child may thus be forestalled (Fonagy, 1998). Serious disturbances of feeding and sleeping, crying and difficulty in bonding continuously confront doctors and health visitors. Many of these can be helped by routine primary care work, but when problems persist, they may be referred to me. It is striking that in this brief work with distressed families large numbers of parents have anxieties about separation and most have experienced traumatic bereavement or loss (Daws, 1993).

Although this work is brief, often one or two meetings only, the method is psychoanalytically based. Problems are thought of as connected with emotions and in the context of the baby's and the parents' history. I ask parents to tell me the problem but then add that in order to help them, I need to understand how the problem has arisen. I ask them for memories of the pregnancy and birth and of how they got together. This may lead on to talking about their own childhoods and their relationship to their parents now. In describing all this, links between ideas often emerge, and parents seem strikingly relieved to make these connections.

Psychosomatic aspects of the work

Doctors and health visitors in the community are struggling every day with body-mind issues. As a psychoanalytically trained worker, I hope to help in understanding the emotional meaning of some patients' symptoms and the feelings aroused in professionals by patients. In families, thoughts about normal development of infants and parents' care are directed first to the baby's *body* and to physical needs. A parent's first duty is simply to keep their baby alive. Stern (1985) has described the interplay between babies and their caretakers and noted that babies need another person in order to experience their own bodies. Babies need the physical mediation of another person to satisfy their hunger or deal with other physical states, such as getting to sleep. Stern says: 'others regulate the infant's experience of somatic state . . . in all such regulations a dramatic shift in neurophysiological state is involved' (p. 103).

In a baby clinic, babies' bodies are examined, as well as attention paid to development and relationships. The weighing scales are important as a focal point for the baby clinic (Daws, 1985). The rationale for parents coming to the clinic can be to have their baby weighed. The baby's body is looked at, appreciated, and measured by parents and professionals. Also apparent is the quality of the mother's ability to protect her infant. Babies are vulnerable in their nakedness when put on the weighing scale and picked up again. We all know the infants' startle reaction when their clothes are taken off. Small babies can look as though they feel they are 'falling to pieces' at this moment. Many mothers intuitively sense this and wrap their baby round by holding with their gaze and with their voice, as well as with their hands. Others cannot do so, and the baby's vulnerability is exposed. All this can be noticed by a receptive health visitor and help her think about what a particular family needs from her. (Incidentally, it is worth noting that an adult, undressing to be examined by the doctor, may be as liable to the startle reaction as any infant.) The weighing scales themselves can also be seen as a kind of 'scales of justice.' This can be a benign process when babies are doing well. However, when there are serious concerns, parents who feel persecuted may split off their own judgement and argue about the accuracy of the scales, leaving professionals alone to worry about the infant's needs. With infants who are failing to thrive, this can be a real danger.

It takes as much skill to stand next to a weighing machine as it does not to talk during a psychotherapy session! The skill of thinking on behalf of the patient is only evident if one says one's thoughts in words, but if one talks too much, reflective thought has no time to grow. Standing doing nothing equally requires skill if it is not to be puzzling and persecuting to the people around. It is legitimised in a busy clinic because all professionals stand at times looking around, sometimes deciding what to do next, sometimes talking to one another. I could be any of these: standing to watch what is going on, or ready for discussion. I must be careful not to get annoyingly in the way of busy staff actually trying to weigh the babies or get to the filing cabinet! If I am too self-contained, it must seem that my observations are for some unexplained private use: if I look too efficiently outgoing, mothers hand me their baby books to check them into the clinic! By watching, I gain what for me is invaluable – seeing a whole range of mothers and babies interact. The time I spend is, of course, usually a few minutes here and there, between sessions with patients, perhaps longer when families fail to turn up. Weekly, my store of impressions of normality and pathology is reinforced so that when someone is referred to me with a problem, I have a background of knowing where this might fit in with what usually happens between parents and babies.

The families who are referred with their baby are often those who seem to remain in a high state of anxiety, in spite of a great deal of supportive work by primary care professionals. There is usually an actual symptom in the baby, such as a feeding or a sleep problem. Often, we then find relationship issues between parents and baby, such as separation problems, perhaps based on earlier bereavements and losses. Some people talk more easily about physical symptoms than about emotions, and McDougall (1986) has popularised the concept of alexythymia (Nemiah & Sifneos, 1970) of people unable to recognise and distinguish their emotions. Parents, in this state of mind, do not *name* their children's emotions, and the children are likely to express feelings through bodily sensations, experiencing physical rather than mental discomfort. Whatever the origin, we must not forget that there has actually been a physical symptom. The baby has *actually* cried with colic, been unable to sleep, is feeding too often, or failing to thrive. Our bodies and minds intertwine, and it does sometimes seem that babies' bodies are affected by the anxieties and traumas in their parents' minds.

A psychoanalytic approach

In this style of work, emotions, relationships, and personal histories are all taken as relevant in thinking about an infant's problem. This is different from the focus of some other therapists working behaviourally or cognitively. Douglas and Richman (1984), for example, state:

> In practice we have found that generally it is not useful to delve back into the past, or into the parents' or the child's psyche to find out the cause of a sleep problem. It is more profitable to concentrate on the here and now of how parents are responding at night-time and how that might affect the sleep patterns.
>
> (p. 47)

By contrast, in my own experience, when families are really listened to, even in brief work, it may enable them to feel that something crucial about them has been understood. They may then be better able to understand and respond to each other and thus deal with their children's problems (Daws, 1993).

Observation and consultation

The child psychotherapist's training begins with the experience of infant observation – seeing an 'ordinary' baby at home, with mother and perhaps other members of the family, for an hour a week for two years (Miller et al.,

1989). The trainee has the chance to see the normal physical, emotional, and social development of an infant. Trainees can also experience the emotions stirred up by this exposure to the intensity of being with a tiny baby, and the drama of the mother-baby relationship. Learning to observe, with respect and with self-containment, is a difficult art. It is also an economical way of learning how to start being a therapist, how to observe what is going on for others in an emotionally heightened situation, to note the feelings stirred up in oneself, to learn how to manage them, and to use these as a source of information, *not* as a key to action. This observing stance is the basis for the consultation that is part of what I as a child psychotherapist can offer the baby clinic.

At the end of the baby clinic, a meeting of health visitors, doctors, and the nurse who has carried out immunisations reviews each attendance, and any worries about a baby and its family are noted. These meetings are a necessary exchange of information; they are also an opportunity to share the experience of the anxieties that have accumulated during the two hours or more of the baby clinic. By being there, I can thus be part of the process where anxieties are picked up and highlighted, or where the group reassures itself that all can be left and reconsidered again next week.

One of my problems is to decide when it is appropriate to help *raise* the anxiety level in colleagues and when to help *settle* it. In general practice, and in the baby clinic, doctors and health visitors are seeing the whole range of the population. In the main they are supporting normality and healthy development. In order for such a clinic to survive, there must be a basic assumption that the anxieties brought constantly are being met, and dealt with, by the routine activities of the clinic.

Parents who have just had a baby are *normally* in a heightened state of emotion: life and death feelings are part of the ordinary state of a baby clinic. Doctors and health visitors have to tolerate the stress of this and evaluate when some of it is out of the ordinary and needs special attention. My focus on anxieties can be a relief to the team, but at other times it can be irritating, and I am felt to pathologise ordinary life events. The professionals also have to cope with the feelings aroused in themselves. This leads to what may be the most helpful contribution that a psychoanalytically trained worker can bring to a primary care team: helping the team to learn to identify the feelings aroused by patients, to manage these feelings, and indeed to use them as a valuable source of information about feelings the patient might have and be unable to tolerate.

Meetings with general practice registrars

As part of this process, there are regular meetings with the GP registrars – doctors in a trainee year. One of the skills of a GP is in assessing what lies behind a patient's request for attention to a particular symptom or condition: 'It's my leg, doctor.' Any illness or symptom implies subtle connections between body and mind. Many patients are longing to be asked about themselves and have a need to be 'known' by their doctor; others are offended by any straying from the obvious task. In this practice, the registrars are well supported by their trainers, but cumulative experience of patients' undefined needs can be overwhelming. One registrar said to me that the meetings were a chance to 'let off steam.' This, in itself, must be useful for a profession that has a high sickness rate (Hale & Hudson, 1992).

In an inner-city practice, there are patients who seem to bring generations of social, relationship, and personal problems to any consultation. When small children from such a family are brought to the surgery, it feels like the opportunity for a 'fresh start.' Young idealistic doctors bring energy to this. They also wish to be realistic, and expectations of what is possible need to be thought about. Airing the feelings of hope, talking of therapeutic zeal and of disappointment, makes it possible to keep on trying. Doctors need to learn to entrust such feelings to each other; on occasion the visiting psychotherapist, by virtue of being an outsider, can be the useful recipient of these feelings. It is, of course, not appropriate for these exchanges to lapse into personal psychotherapy sessions; they must be confined to the medical task. Doctors, whether in training or experienced, have to learn to work fast. Corney (1996) has pointed out that doctors do not 'have the luxury of time to reflect on their practice.' Any psychotherapist working with GPs learns to speed up and report back fast! However, it may be that, as Corney suggests, 'if doctors took more time for reflection, it could enable them to function more effectively and feel more supported' (p. 137).

Meetings with health visitors

I also have regular meetings with the health visitors in addition to many short informal discussions during baby clinics. We sometimes talk about cases they might wish to refer to me. More often, we will talk about a case that is perplexing or, even more likely, irritating or angering them. We talk about where these feelings come from, about how some people provoke anger and rejection as they go through life. A health visitor who understands that the parent may be re-enacting the rejection she has experienced in her childhood will not be put off. The mother may start to feel understood and supported for the first time and may, in turn, manage the baby's feelings better.

I may be able to back the health visitor in keeping going with the parents who need this help most but turn it away. Because they are available to *all* families of new babies, health visitors are able to support families through the uncertain first days of getting to know a new baby, and how to care for it. When health visitors give expert advice to families, it may also feel as though they are symbolically 'parenting' these families, especially when there is a lack of such support. The beneficial effect of this is unquantifiable. When families are in emotional trouble, the health visitor, who already has a relationship built on many meetings and much knowledge, is in the best position to help. This implies caseloads that allow time to work with the families that do need more attention, rather than having to refer them on to designated specialist health visitors dealing only with identified problems or to other professionals.

Postnatal depression

In this practice, general practitioners and health visitors alike have always been sensitive to the emotional state of women who have recently had babies, but postnatal depression is a condition that is difficult to diagnose. First, most women feel *really* depressed only when alone with their babies. In the presence, even briefly, of an interested health visitor they may feel cared for. On the other hand, those who are most severely depressed can be so flat, elusive, and dismissing of any approach that it is easy for the health visitor to feel unwanted and, in turn, not be readily available for the mother.

Cox's study on postnatal depression included giving a brief questionnaire on their emotional state to women who had just given birth (Cox et al., 1987). This Edinburgh Postnatal Depression Scale is effective in detecting depression, but its use is still controversial. Some of the most clinically inspired health visitors feel that the discovery of the depression through the scale creates a barrier between themselves and the mother and that the real discovery of depression needs to take place during a spontaneous, open-ended conversation between health visitor and mother. The questionnaire can then be used to back up clinical intuition, and Seeley (2001) says that the scale is only as good as the person interpreting it. Timing and context are thus crucial in sensitive use of the scale. However, the Edinburgh scale did alert us to the prevalence of postnatal depression. Following this, Holden and colleagues suggested that eight weekly counselling sessions by a health visitor is an effective way of helping postnatally depressed women (Holden et al., 1989). This is an important advance in treatment and underlines the crucial part that health visitors play in the primary care facilities of this country.

The counselling function of general practitioners and health visitors

I believe that one of my most helpful functions is to back the primary care team to be 'braver' in taking on the difficulties in relationships that many families have. The long-term relationship families can have with their GP and health visitor is in itself a model for parents. Referrals to specialists (including myself) must be carefully considered lest they puncture this attachment.

How, therefore, does a health visitor or a general practitioner who has such a long-term relationship with an individual or a family do some serious 'counselling' work and then go back to the usual brief consultations? The latter are captured in the title of the book *Six Minutes for the Patient* (Balint & Norrell, 1973), the authors of which describe the brief, intense, and close contact, which they call a 'flash,' that can happen even within an ordinary consultation between doctor and patient. Such a meeting may lead to an offer of a longer appointment, which has more of the nature of a counselling session. I believe that through just one, or perhaps a few, such meetings, a patient can feel that they are really known about by their doctor or health visitor and that this remains a reference point when the more routine relationship is resumed. It is important that this process does remain under control, otherwise the general practitioner's constant fear of endless need becoming unleashed could become a reality.

So, how much can, or should, health visitors and general practitioners themselves take part in counselling? Professionals, even without a psychotherapy or counselling training, can extend their scope of working. Zalidis (1994) describes a contained way in which doctors can look at the here and now relationship with their patients:

> The doctor's increased understanding of the relationship with his patients enables him to become more tolerant and more receptive to what his patients are telling him, without necessarily attempting to challenge their defences, or make interpretations. The resulting improved relationship with the doctor can lead to a therapeutic change in the patient.
>
> (p. 182)

Elder (1987) has pointed out the emotional dangers of attempting too much. He says that general practitioners

> hoping to make their patients better will soon be exhausted and disillusioned. Doctors in general practice have to learn to live with their patients in a much more unchanging world than often both would wish. The frustrations of this has to be borne, just as uncertainty also has to be, in order to allow other possible changes to occur.
>
> (p. 54)

He asks to what extent to these two worlds – the doctor's and the patient's – meet in moments of understanding.

The key to understanding is *listening*, and there are two elements to this: first, listening to patients, giving them time for what they have to say, and taking note of how they say it; second, attending to the feelings stirred up in oneself as a worker and seeing what information these feelings bring to bear on the patient. This approach can be taught by working jointly with a referring professional. For example, I saw a mother with two hyperactive toddlers, together with their health visitor. Hyperactivity, like many other presenting problems, may be a sign of a relationship difficulty; it is necessary first to hear in detail about the nature of the problem. The mother told us how out of control she experienced her two boys as being. It also became evident that she was very angry with them for this behaviour, and she rarely looked at them as she spoke. It is important not to go directly to solutions of the symptom. In talking with this mother, we soon heard a story of losses in her life, and it seemed that she had been severely postnatally depressed and was still suffering from depression. She cried as she told her story, and the health visitor put her arm around her. The two children quietened down as they played, seeming relieved that their mother had had a chance to unburden herself, possibly for the first time. Perhaps they perceived us as looking after her and could relax their 'responsibility' for her. She was able to think about whether her children's 'hyperactive' rushing about was their attempt to produce some life in their flat, dispirited mother (Murray & Cooper, 1997). As she began to feel sympathetic to their predicament, she was able to watch their play, and the children, in turn, responded to this interest, showing her the small toy cars and animals they were using.

Afterwards, the health visitor told me that she was impressed with how much the mother had been able to confide in us. Then she confessed: 'At first I couldn't stand the silences.' I thought, 'What silences?' Compared to a psychotherapy session, it had been all talk! In order to communicate emotions as well as thoughts, we have to use more than just words. All sorts of nonverbal signs pass from one person to another, and some silences may be an essential part of this.

Silences are necessary, but long ones are to be avoided: a few seconds may be enough. What is important is for the patient sometimes to be the one to break the silence. Psychoanalytic method is based *on free association* – that is, patients letting their minds move freely from one thought to another, to see where thoughts lead. It would be pretentious and confusing to use this method in ordinary professional exchanges. Patients naturally expect a conversation. But it can be very rewarding to allow patients the space sometimes to say what comes into *their* minds, following what *they* have just said, rather than workers breaking the train of thought with their own words.

Working like this is difficult because much of what we say to patients can be to keep them quiet, to *stop* the flow of what they might say next, especially if they are depressed or disturbed in some way. For example, postnatally depressed mothers may, given the chance, relate shocking thoughts of anxiety, anger, self-hatred, hatred of the baby or partner, disturbing dreams, fears of damage that has, or might, happen. The urge to cheer people up or to keep things under control rather than to hear the content of depressing or upsetting thoughts can be overwhelming. So anyone who extends their range of competence, becoming more of a counsellor, needs *supervision* as they get to grips with what happens when patients are encouraged to talk. McLeod (1988) has emphasised the need for supervision for all counsellors, and Corney (1993) has pointed out that training improves outcome.

Clinical applications

In the baby clinic, where does the need for specific clinical work by the psychotherapist fit in? There are various reasons why a referral may be justified. First, there are some parents who can make use of intensive time away from the known primary care workers when issues can be explored in depth. This is separate protected time with some privacy, though not necessarily confidential from the referrer.

The referral process itself, where the GP or health visitor suggests to the family that they could see a psychotherapist, can feel either like concerned care or as a rejection. I treasure a remark made by one GP about a too-hasty referral to me by a colleague, saying that the patient had been 'mugged' by the therapy!

Next are the cases where anxiety remains after medical needs have been properly attended to. In one referral the mother of a six-week-old baby told me that she had called out four doctors over the weekend because the baby had a cold. Each doctor had suggested to her that she should see me. They had all sensed her anxiety level, but it turned out that this anxiety had a very real basis. She had had various losses and traumas, including a stillbirth. Any small ailment triggered fears of serious loss. In such a case, putting a patient's fears into words is, of course, helpful in itself, and going through an actual traumatic experience may help recovery from it; the work also needs to take on the personal meaning for an individual of such events. Any parent will naturally have ambivalent feelings towards their baby. When the baby is especially precious, it can be hard to own the hostile part of these feelings. Unacknowledged ambivalence can be one of the clues to excessive anxiety. A therapist who can bear hearing painful experiences and thoughts that the patient feels to be shocking may help anxiety move to a more manageable level.

Paradoxically, it can sometimes be useful to see families even when there are many problems besetting them, and it would appear that there is too much going on for psychotherapy in itself to be effective. Meeting the family face to face does at least give me a vivid experience of their problems and of the effect a 'heart-sink' family can have on a would-be helpful professional. I can then share the feelings of the primary care team as we discuss how to manage such long-term difficult families. It can also be realistic to use specialist time to attempt to reach, in the familiar surroundings of their health centre, a few families not normally thought likely to use this work. The attempt in itself stretches my technique; it may help some deprived people to feel that their doctor and health visitor have not given up on them, and might stir them into more self-awareness and responsibility. I often think that if all referrals were 'suitable cases for treatment,' we would all be missing an opportunity to see who might be able to use the chance to think differently about themselves.

Case study: 'Harry'

I now give a brief example of a case where the symptom in the baby could be seen to connect with experiences in the family. A family was referred for a severe sleep problem in their nine-month-old baby, Harry.

When I met the family, father, mother, and baby all gazed at me seriously as I invited them into the consulting room. The parents relaxed as we made our introductions. I remarked that the baby looked worried. Father said that he was usually a smiley baby. I said that perhaps they were all a bit worried about coming to talk about problems with a strange person and that it showed how sensitive he was to their feelings. Both parents agreed. By commenting at the start on the level of anxiety that seemed apparent to me, I was setting the scene for a focus on emotional issues in the consultation.

With this clue of the baby's sensitivity, I was first told about the presenting problem: that this baby could only go to sleep while on the breast, and that he woke many times during the night and each time had to be fed back to sleep by his mother. During the day, he did not need to be fed so much but was very distressed if his mother was out of his sight.

I then asked about the pregnancy and birth and of the process of getting together in the early weeks. As the story unfolded, I asked about the parents' own childhoods and tried to make links. In this family, one piece of information was overwhelming. There had been a traumatic event at the birth of the baby: at the end of labour, the mother had suffered an amniotic fluid embolism and had become unconscious. There was then a night of endeavour to save her life, and she was told that if a particular consultant who recognised her serious condition had not happened to be there, she might well have died. She told me of this doctor calling her name as she recovered consciousness – it felt as though he was calling her back to life.

As I considered this dramatic story, the parents told me more about the baby's waking during the night. They also had a nine-year-old son, who, they felt, had no problems. I also learnt that the mother's parents had both died when she was in her adolescence. I remarked that she knew how unbearable it was to lose a parent, and perhaps she needed to keep her baby especially close to her, when he had also so nearly lost her. Many cases of severe sleep problems have had a serious loss in the family's history (Daws, 1993). It seemed clear that her anxiety was also communicating itself to the baby in a way that prevented him from switching off into sleep.

I then happened to ask her whether she had nightmares about her near-death. She said that she had not, and that she herself barely slept. It occurred to me that her experience of being called back to life by the doctor had made her equate sleep with death. It sounded as though she had to stay awake so as not to lapse into death. She agreed, but then told me that her difficulty in sleeping dated from her father's death. He had died of a heart attack and she had found him dead in bed in the morning. She had always felt that if she had woken earlier and gone to him sooner, he would not have died. When her mother had died a few years later, she became responsible for younger siblings and similarly felt that she had to stay 'on guard' on their behalf. This mother's own difficulty in sleeping is, therefore, multiply determined.

I next discovered that father had a different approach to sleep. Although a committed and involved father, he could not help his wife with the night-time problems, as he slept so deeply that he did not wake when the baby cried. It then emerged that his own mother had never woken to attend to him as a baby, his father having been the one to respond. Here again, we see evidence of the impact of attachment relationships on sleep.

In this first meeting, the baby was sitting in his buggy, gravely staring at me. Father then released him and held him on his knee. As the baby started to grizzle, father made as though to hand him to mother. I said, 'What would happen if you kept hold of him?' Father said, 'He'll probably start to cry,' but he turned Harry towards him and swung him in the air. Harry chuckled, and resettled down again on his father's lap. In fact, he stayed there for the rest of the hour of our meeting. It gave us the opportunity to think about how the whole family had begun to believe that only mother could soothe Harry but that perhaps his father could also do it. When fathers are able to share in the comforting of their baby, it not only lessens the strains on the mother, the father may also gain some authority in stopping the baby from an endless exploitation of the mother. In this method of parent-infant psychotherapy, using the evidence in the room of small examples of behaviour enables the therapist and family to notice and think about their usual way of interacting and the philosophy behind this.

The next time, mother came with Harry on her own because of father's shift work. Father had started to spend more time with the baby. Harry's sleeping had improved a little, and the two parents were actively thinking about how to get him out of their bed and into his cot. Parents first of all need to have their own anxieties acknowledged and also recount their different childhood histories. Sometimes a great deal of conflicting experience needs to be talked about before parents can be helped in getting together about the sleep problem. I usually find that the baby then quickly responds, and sleeps better.

In this case, it seemed as important to concentrate on mother's sleeping problem as that of her baby. She had told me that after the trauma of her embolism, she had become 'pessimistic' about everything. I felt that her use of the word was quite appropriate: it was not the same as being depressed. I commented that by never getting long-enough cycles of sleep, she was missing out on the way that dreaming restores optimism. Hartman (1973) has stated that the ability to maintain an optimistic mood, energy, and self-confidence requires not just sleep itself but, specifically, REM sleep, which comes at the end of each sleep cycle. Similarly, she was missing out on the post-traumatic recuperative process that dreams and nightmares could have provided. Palombo (1978) has talked of the integrating function of dreaming and assimilating experiences into long-term memory. So, ironically, the stresses that led to her lack of sleep were perpetuated by the effects of the sleeplessness.

I believe that sorting out experiences by talking can fulfil some of the missing functions of dreaming. I also suggested that physical exercise, walking, swimming, and so on without the baby could get this mother into the sort of free-associating state where she could lose her watchfulness and thus sleep better and allow her baby also to relax into sleep. This reflective approach was perhaps helpful to a family striving to recover from trauma. When the work finished, the baby was sleeping better.

Conclusion

The value of a child psychotherapist working in the baby clinic of a general practice is twofold. First is the clinical work of seeing families with infants. Many of the common problems of infancy such as those with sleeping and feeding have an emotional basis. Many families also come openly with relationship and attachment issues. Such families can often be helped within a few meetings.

Second, this clinical exposure can be put to wider use. Our contact with patients gives us confirmation of theoretical ideas about individual internal processes and family functioning, and particularly about the recognising and use of feelings stirred up in ourselves by our patients. The real application of the knowledge gained is in sharing it with doctors or health visitors who see many more families than is possible for us.

In CAMHS clinics referrals, even if self-made, have a formal structure, and cases can be 'closed.' GPs and health visitors, in contrast, have an open-ended relationship with their patients, or clients. As evaluation in all aspects of medical work becomes imperative, a psychotherapist can perhaps back the primary care team in continuing to recognise the importance of the emotional and psychosomatic aspects of their work, and in keeping going over years of dealing with the cumulative experience of seeing patients with undefined needs. Ongoing consultation with an appreciative outside colleague can help the team both with rigorous standards of keeping to the task and with higher self-appreciation of the value of the work.

References

Balint, E., Courtenay, M., Elder, A., Hull, S., & Julian, P. (1993). *The Doctor, the Patient and the Group: Balint Revisited*. London: Routledge.

Balint, E., & Norrell, J. (Eds.). (1973). *Six Minutes for the Patient*. London: Tavistock.

Balint, M. (1957). *The Doctor, His Patient and the Illness*. London: Pitman.

Brook, A. (1978). 'An aspect of community mental health: Consultative work with general practice teams'. *Health Trends*, 10 (2): 37–40.

Corney, R. (1993). 'Studies of the effectiveness of counselling in general practice'. In: R. Corney & R. Jenkins (Eds.), *Counselling in General Practice*. London: Routledge.

Corney, R. (1996). 'Studies of the effectiveness of counselling in general practice'. In: R. Corney & R. Jenkins (Eds.), *Counselling in General Practice*. London: Routledge.

Cox, J. L., Holden, J. M., & Sagovsky, R. (1987). 'Detection of postnatal depression'. *British Journal of Psychiatry*, 150: 782–6.

Daws, D. (1985). 'Standing next to the weighing scales'. *Journal of Child Psychotherapy*, 11: 77–85.

Daws, D. (1993). *Through the Night: Helping Parents and Sleepless Infants*. London: Free Association Books.

Daws, D. (1995). 'Psychotherapy in the community'. In: J. Trowell & M. Bower (Eds.), *The Emotional Needs of Young Children and Their Families*. London: Routledge.

Douglas, J., & Richman, N. (1984). *My Child Won't Sleep*. Harmondsworth: Penguin.

Elder, A. (1986). 'Psychotherapy in general practice'. In: H. Maxwell (Ed.), *Psychotherapy: An Outline for Trainee Psychiatrists, Medical Students and Practitioners*. London: Whurr.

Elder, A. (1987). 'Moments of change'. In: A. Elder & O. Samuel (Eds.), *While I'm Here, Doctor: A Study of the Doctor Patient Relationship*. London: Tavistock Press.

Fonagy, P. (1998). 'Prevention, the appropriate target of infant psychotherapy'. *Infant Mental Health Journal*, 19: 124–50.

Hale, R., & Hudson, L. (1992). 'The Tavistock study of young doctors: Report of the pilot phase'. *British Journal of Hospital Medicine*, 47: 452–64.

Hartman, E. (1973). *The Functions of Sleep*. New Haven, CT: Yale University Press.

Holden, J. H., Sagovsky, R., & Cox, J. L. (1989). 'Counselling in general practice settings: Controlled study of health visitor intervention in treatment of postnatal depression'. *British Medical Journal*, 298: 223–6.

Launer, J. (1994). 'Psychotherapy in the general practitioner surgery: Working with and without a secure therapeutic frame'. *British Journal of Psychotherapy*, 11: 120–6.

McDougall, J. (1986). *Theatres of the Mind*. London: Free Association Books.

McLeod, J. (1988). 'The work of counsellors in general practice'. In: *Occasional Paper 37*. London: Royal College of General Practitioners.

Miller, L., Rustin, M., Rustin, M., & Shuttleworth, J. (Eds.). (1989). *Closely Observed Infants*. London: Duckworth.

Murray, L., & Cooper, P. J. (Eds.). (1997). *Postnatal Depression and Child Development*. London: Guilford Press.

Nemiah, J. C., & Sifneos, P. E. (1970). 'Psychosomatic illness: A problem in communication'. *Psychotherapy and Psychosomatics*, 18 (1–6): 154–60.

Palombo, S. (1978). *Dreaming and Memory*. New York: Basic Books.

Seeley, S. (2001). 'Strengths and limitations of the Edinburgh postnatal depression scale'. In: *Postnatal Depression and Maternal Mental Health: A Public Health Priority*. London: Community Practitioners and Health Visitors Association Conference Proceedings.

Stern, D. (1985). *The Interpersonal World of the Infant*. New York: Basic Books.

Zalidis, S. (1994). 'The value of emotional awareness in general practice'. In: A. Erskine & D. Judd (Eds.), *The Imaginative Body*. London: Whurr.

3 Psychoanalysis and the public service

Can they inspire each other?

Originally given as a paper at the Tavistock Scientific Meeting in June 2000, and at the Montreal WAIMH Congress in July 2000. The version appearing here has been abbreviated.

In January 1998, David Campbell gave a scientific lecture entitled 'Ideas Which Divide the Tavistock: What Are They Really About?' I thought I'd like to do something like that and I hope that stimulating further thought was, in part, his intention. He said, 'Systems theory has taught me that any group, such as a family or staff group, needs diversity and heterogeneity to survive. We need diversity at the Tavistock and we have it, but I think there is more we could do to utilise its potential for our growth and development.'

David was looking at the diversity *within* the Tavistock. I am assuming much common ground and want to consider our need for influences *outside* the Tavistock to stimulate our creativity.

Firstly, most of us training as psychotherapists have come from working in another profession, social work, teaching, nursing medicine, etc. We have discovered a need to get more deeply into the difficulties we have been trying to understand, but we are in fact also bringing much knowledge to this new discipline.

Yet bringing together different ways of working, and the institutions that house them, is not always an easy process. Some years after qualifying from the Tavistock as a child psychotherapist, I began working at the Day Unit in Daleham Gardens, and its parent clinic, the Child Guidance Training Centre. This was another kind of diversity. We prided ourselves on being the oldest training clinic in the country, and both we and the Tavistock defined ourselves through our differences. The merger of the CGTC with the Tavistock took place in 1985, with a further merger between it and the children and parents department a couple of years later to create C&F. This rapprochement, mostly forgotten now, was very painful at the time – much that had been thought naturally essential had to be changed. The process of getting together was exhausting – my

DOI: 10.4324/b23125-4

husband said that for months I looked grey with tiredness when I got home. I don't think I was the only one. But we were eventually revitalised by this exposure to each other and much creativity came from it. In a moment I will consider some of our motivation for work in the public service – but working with colleagues must be a large and compelling part of it.

It is worth considering some of the negative connotations associated with working in the public service. It is not necessary to remind anyone working in this building that government upholding of clinical standards can be experienced not just as intrusive but as actually making the work it is intended to promote impossible to perform, that thinking about clinical work can be negated by bureaucratic misunderstanding. Furthermore, taking responsibility for a wider concept of mental health can make an individual clinician feel guilty and impotent that they can only take on a certain number of patients and that they will never get through the waiting list of what seems like an entire population needing help with emotional life from the likes of us.

So what is the motivation to work in such an apparently stressful situation? A Tavistock patient, a young mother, recently said to me, 'I know you really care about me because I don't pay you.' I pointed out that I was paid to see her and it was part of my job. We could then look at the fact that I might nevertheless care about her welfare. In transference terms, we could also think about her feelings about how and to what extent her parents or others had cared for her in the past, or do so now. In working with children in care, one of the most painful realisations was that they were always cared for by people whose job it was to do so. You could say that these professional carers had chosen to do it, and that these children's parents had chosen not to. But the children's experience was always of someone being on duty to look after them.

So is one motivation to *appear* to be generous? In fact, we are spared the burden of personal generosity by the mediation of the State – we are also employees, we are one part of an enormous public service, the largest employer in the country. We are therefore beneficiaries of the system. It might seem naïve to talk about idealism in public service, but in the course of teaching and discussing my work in other countries without an NHS, I have been made aware of the difference in atmosphere when there is not an over-arching system to belong to. There is no obligation to reach difficult kinds of patients, let alone the ones who can't pay. The boundaries between professions are easier to cross, when we all belong to the same system, and communications on behalf of patients are possible to make. Above all, in public service, it is a relief not to be solely responsible for the best of one's aspirations – to be able to project them into a system or an institution that one can then belong to.

As I have mentioned elsewhere, describing my father's work as a GP, the informal system of doctors balancing private fee-paying patients with those seen for free was replaced by the creation of the NHS. This gesture towards equality by doctors in this country must have been part of the motivation for setting up the NHS. Public policies replaced individual commitment.

Some of my patients in a general practice would not manage coming to see someone other than in their own family doctor's surgery. I sometimes feel that helping these disturbed people, getting to know their thought processes and emotions, gives me a lot personally. More painful is when these encounters are both an effort to support parenting, and also part of an assessment of whether these parents are really able to care for their babies. It is an honour when parents can, at least in part, trust you with benign intent on behalf of their baby and perhaps themselves in these circumstances. It is only in public service that you have such an opportunity and this is my first example of public service work inspiring psychoanalytic thinking. You really need to think about the soundness of your theories when people's lives depend on it. This includes attachment theory, ideas about the internalised influence of experience, about the possible mediating effect of new attachment to a new baby. With this, you can be a useful part of a team, making crucial decisions.

It is very satisfying when psychoanalytic ideas make sense to ordinary people – ideas about projective processes, about intergenerational influences, about transference, or repression. When such ideas are received as common sense, I think it gives them a new vitality.

A patient told me that her friend, a former patient, had said of me, 'She's good, she works fast.' An unusual compliment for a psychotherapist. I think the need for brief work can make one pull out the essence of analytic technique.

What can be called psychoanalytic? Child psychotherapists undoubtedly have a psychoanalytic training – personal psychoanalysis, three supervised intensive cases, and a whole lot more. However, much of our work is not with individual patients seen several times a week. We see children once a week, we see families, we do brief therapy, we work with the professional network. There has been recent discussion, some apologetic, often proclaiming the value of all this as *applied* psychoanalysis. It is perhaps more accurate to use the term 'psychoanalytic thinking' to describe a stance from which to promote action. Psychoanalysis is indeed about reflection and self-reflection, what Bollas and Sundelson call 'psychoanalytic quiet' – but this does not need to imply non-action.

In the Cherry Orchard, you see the Russian custom of sitting down for a moment before undertaking a journey. If we take the mental health of the community seriously, we need to sit down, or even lie down, reflectively before making the journey to a wider section of the population. This could be called psychoanalytic thinking in action.

We Infant Mental Health specialists work alongside doctors and health visitors for ordinary pregnancies, births, infant development, and the support of parent-infant attachment. We learn from them as they learn from us. We also learn much from our intimate involvement with ordinary people in the community. The therapist's consultative work with the doctors and health visitors supports a psychodynamic approach. A therapist can help colleagues to think before acting and be braver in taking on emotions, psychosomatic links, and transferences. Such consultation is not teaching about interventions but standing uncertainty and emotional distress without jumping to active strategies.

Two crucial points come in here. Firstly, that this work about emotions with infants and their families is of the utmost importance. Here is the chance to make things go well or badly for life. Work with families with new babies, and with the network around them, is *the* way to underpin the mental health of the whole country.

Secondly is really the main point of my talk. Only in public service do we have a responsibility for everyone who needs a particular kind of work. We also have access to all these people. This can either paralyse us into immobility, as I suggested earlier, or liberate us into thinking how to modify our technique in a way that remains true to its principles and has wider application.

Part 2

Parent-infant psychotherapy and infant mental health

4   Parent-infant psychotherapy

The baby in the consulting room

Originally published in the Journal of the British Association of Psychotherapists
(2002, Vol. 40).

Introduction

This article is a pragmatic one – I am writing mainly about working with actual
babies in the room in parent-infant psychotherapy. However, it also gives us
the opportunity to think about the metaphor of the infant in an adult patient's
mind. In thinking how to conceptualise the difference between adult psychoanalytic psychotherapy and parent-infant work, I realised that in work with families we deal with the realities before they are translated into metaphors. Breasts
and shit are everywhere! Babies are actually fed, their nappies are changed, in
the room. These basic bodily functions and the emotions that accompany them
are experienced directly between the baby and its parents; the therapist is an
observer, and not necessarily the *recipient* of transference communications.
What she observes of course includes parents' perceptions of their baby, influenced by transferences from their own past experiences.

More than 60 years ago Ella Sharpe made similar connections in her article
'Psycho-Physical Problems Revealed in Language: An Examination of Metaphor' (1940). Noting that 'No word is metaphysical without its first having
been physical,' she says that when listening to patients the search must be for
'the physical basis and experience from which metaphysical speech springs.'
Her theory is that 'metaphor can only evolve in language or in the arts when
bodily orifices become controlled.' Examples of such metaphors used by her
adult patients include:

> I've wandered off the point and can't find it again.
> I've lost sight of what I came for.
> It's the way I set about things that's wrong.[1]

DOI: 10.4324/b23125-6

Sharpe suggests that difficulties in physical and mental manipulation in adult life, such as awkwardness, 'doing things the wrong way,' or an inability to keep to the point or to concentrate, have their origins in suckling experiences. When these have been traumatic, the patient unconsciously expects a repetition of this. Likewise, there are metaphors about anal and urethral matters such as:

> I am sodden with despair.
> I'm depressed, I suppose I'm making heavy weather of my troubles.
> I feel I've landed myself in a mess.
> I've a fear of letting myself go altogether.

She says that a spontaneous metaphor is the epitome of a forgotten experience: 'It can reveal a present-day physical condition which is based upon an original psycho-physical experience.' She continues, 'The metaphors of depression denote the zero hour, exhaustion and immobility, giving us the physical setting which first accompanied the psychical feelings; prolonged crying, bed-wetting, loneliness and exhaustion.' Other metaphors give pictures of futile activity, achievement of no goal, continual thwarting and obstructing of the self. I would say that parent-infant work takes us very close to these raw physical settings and feelings out of which the metaphors, dear to psychoanalysis, arise.

Parent-infant therapy, and particularly *brief* therapy, is, appropriately enough, one of the largest growth areas in psychoanalytically based work. This work is also perhaps a meeting point for psychoanalytic and family therapy concepts.

Tom Main, one of the British 'Independents,' said of psychoanalysis that sitting behind a couch five times a week was only one of its applications (personal communication to Eric Rayner and others). With that definition in mind, one need not be shy in thinking of the dramatic and eventful meetings with parents and their infants as equally one of its applications.

My work in parent-infant psychotherapy has been at the Under Fives Counselling Service at the Tavistock Clinic and still continues at a baby clinic in the James Wigg Practice in Kentish Town Health Centre. At both places, the work is with families about difficulties in their infants' development. Many cases are referred as sleeping or feeding problems; in addition some parents will come openly talking about their difficulty in making a relationship with their baby.

I am going to argue that this work is *psychoanalytically based* although it is usually very brief, not more than four to six sessions. It is the approach of taking in and reflecting on what parents tell me, so that an understanding and integrative process begins in my mind, and similarly can take over in theirs. I look together with parents at their baby, noting the baby's uniqueness and so helping them to stand outside fixed ways of thinking and reacting. Although some of the success of this work derives from the experience of seeing many families with such problems, it cannot be done in a routine way – the impact of each family's stress and bewilderment must be received afresh each time.

One of the mechanisms that operate here is that *projections* that have been spat out and that have bounced back and forwards unowned between parents and infants are perhaps rerouted through the therapist. Her ability to receive these feelings and to think about them has a transforming effect. Feelings are commented on, acknowledged and may change. In psychoanalytic thinking, we also assume that many different facets of people's lives interlink with one symptom or disturbance – that is, they are *overdetermined*. With an infant's sleep problem this is certainly so. It need not be daunting to take this on board in brief therapy. My principal hypothesis is that for the therapist to gather in, with the parents, all the relevant aspects of a baby's life and its relationship to them, within the brief framework of the consultation, is itself therapeutic (Daws, 1989).

With this in mind, the method that I use is to combine three different elements. First, there is a questioning about the details of the baby's timetable: as I ask for the precise details of day and night, a vivid picture builds up in my mind of what actually happens in this family and their assumptions of what should happen. The questions themselves sometimes begin to clarify a confused situation as the parents both let me know and think about the implications of the questions. Second, there is a free-ranging inquiry into memories of the pregnancy, birth, and early weeks: I tell parents that I need to know the baby's life story to make sense of what is happening now. Third, I ask about the parents' relationship with one another and with their own parents, so that we see the family context of this particular baby. In every interview, I have in mind very specific information to collect. However, no two interviews are the same. The order and the nature of my questions are always different, dependent, I hope, on picking up the special and unique links in each family's story.

The parents I see have usually been offered much advice already and often feel they have 'tried everything.' What I give them in the first place is simple – ordinary psychoanalytic free-floating attention. As they tell their story, unconscious threads draw together and connections emerge. Because I do not at once offer solutions, they are less likely to react negatively. They are left able to free associate – that is, let their minds lead freely from one related theme to another. They may perceive me as interested, receptive, and capable of holding on to a great deal of information. In this setting, it is striking how parents can convey economically much focused information. It seems as though all ordinary parents have a 'story' to tell about their baby as dramatic and as moving as any work of literature. What is also communicated, and confirmed by my interest, is the uniqueness of each baby and its family.

Parent-infant work is notable for its activity. Enactments are everywhere. Even the way in which families come into the room and settle themselves down, or, as they leave, the length of time it takes to withdraw their infantile transference to the therapist as they slowly put on the baby's outdoor clothes, is worth an article in itself. The timing of sessions must allow for this process as a legitimate part of the work, not as an inconvenient side-effect. During the course of meetings, babies cling to their mothers and feed; they get down, move away, and play; they approach the therapist as the parents feel freer; they cry as painful conflicts are touched on by the adults.

The nature of patients' thinking

One major aim of this work is to consider not just *what* patients think but *how* they think it. In brief work, it is of course impossible to alter the nature of thinking processes. But spotting how a problem is thought about, and how it is described, is vital. There are striking connections between the *description* of the problem and the problem itself.

Sleep problems

With sleep disturbances, I start by letting parents tell me in their own way what the problem is so that I do not lose the particular flavour of what they feel is wrong and its origin. I also hope to experience the predominant emotion with which parents begin their story. Once I have begun to ask questions, I am perhaps felt to be looking after them and intense emotions often subside. Whatever emotions come out strongly in these first few moments are perhaps the same as what the baby feels is directed towards him during his sleepless nights, be it anger, anxiety, or responsible concern. After the parents have told me the problem, I explain that I would like to ask them questions about the baby and the family in general, so that we can discover what links there may be – starting with questions of detail, such as the physical placing of cots and beds and who sleeps with who in each room. I then feel free to get into the general area of family relationships.

Separation problems

Simplistically speaking, the problem for a mother in getting a baby to sleep is the basic act of putting the baby down – that is, of separating herself from her baby and the baby from her. It can be as difficult for the mother to do without the baby as it is the other way around. I have, however, become aware of how many parents these days keep their babies very close to them, by day and by night, for the first months or even longer. In fact, it does seem that there is a biological imperative for this closeness, which in itself aids attachment. Some of these parents find that their baby has difficulty in getting to sleep; many do not. It seems that there is an ability in some parents and babies to enjoy their closeness, and, at the same time, to let go of each other emotionally, enough for each to be free to go to sleep. Other parents and babies come to experience such closeness as a mutual torment of intrusiveness, and no one is able to sleep long and deeply. They seem also to get caught in the closeness and become unable to think about how to get more separate from each other. There are two important issues here. First, *all* babies need closeness and intimacy with their parents to develop a sense of themselves as individuals, as well as a sense of themselves in relation to other people. Second, all babies need at appropriate moments to take steps away from their parents, both literally and metaphorically, in order to begin to grow.

When a family is able to discuss such issues, allowing the therapist as the outsider to have some new ideas of what might be helpful, it shows that the family is ready for change. One such thought is that the use of 'transitional objects' is part of the process by which babies manage some of the first steps of separation (Winnicott, 1971). For instance, when I ask if the baby has a teddy bear, I may be told that she has several cuddly toys. When I suggest that *one* significant toy could be important, parents may be able to create a shared idea with the baby that a particular toy has a job to do. Often, of course, blankets, dummies, or the baby's own thumb may become the source of satisfaction that allows separation from the mother, at the same time as being a link or memory. Parents and babies are able to move on to such solutions when the emotions involved in the original problem have been sufficiently attuned to.

Attunement and dreaming

Attunement and the failure of it is one of our themes. In fact, the hard work of this method of therapy comes from the need for the therapist to be in touch appropriately with each set of individuals. In order to change something, it is necessary to know what it is first. A family comes in a certain state of mind about their child and his sleep problem. It is necessary for the worker to know and be in touch with this state of mind.

The worker who offers this receptivity is assailed by a jumble of information, emotion, and memories. At first I thought of this bombardment just as an unfortunate way of behaving by people who are short of sleep. Hartmann (1973) states that

> sleep and probably D-sleep or REM sleep specifically, may have a restorative function with respect to symptoms of focussed attention (especially the ability to focus on one item while ignoring others) and to maintain an optimistic mood, energy and self-confidence.

From this we would indeed expect parents deprived by their babies of sleep to be short of such attributes. In time, however, I came to recognise such consultations as being often the ones that promised most resolution. It requires the use of another set of ideas to work out how this comes about. Palombo (1978) describes the function of dreams as assimilating memories of the day into settled long-term memory. He says that 'the dream itself . . . and not merely the interpretation of the dream – plays a positive integrating role in normal emotional development.' I see one of the main uses of the consultations as being akin to dream work, for parents nearly always come in a distressed state with a confused mass of information. What happens in the dream work by the process of assimilation also happens in these consultations with parents: the information they bring to the therapist is brought together during the consultation. Kaplan-Solms and Solms's (2000: 46) recent work develops the connection between abstraction and dreams, also suggesting that an important function is in addressing conflicts.

In work on attachment are ideas that link up with this. Mary Main (Main et al., 1985) has noticed that *the manner* in which parents talk about their relationships with their own parents enables prediction on how they get on with their babies. She describes how parents who are themselves insecure in their attachments are *incoherent* in talking about their childhood experiences. The parents I have seen have lost much of their time for dreaming. I perhaps allow them to start to think and then to dream.

Bion (1962) has described how the mother's thinking about her baby enables him to deal with his confused emotional experiences in a way that enables the baby to start thinking and dreaming. I would add that the mother's dreaming is part of this process. Dreams can be a way of anticipating progress before it has been openly achieved, not as a form of 'prophecy' but as an acknowledgement of mental work. Parents' dreams may herald progress in dealing with the problems between them and their children. One father dreamed that his little son, Stanley (who could not yet talk), asked him, 'Why don't you show me how to get to sleep?' This released into consciousness memories that helped father connect what was happening now with similar problems between his own father and himself. This dream thus linked the past with the present, reminding father of his own childhood difficulties, and apparently informing him that *his* father's failure to help him was part of the background of his own failure to help his son now. However, I think Stanley's words in the dream, 'Why don't you show me how to get to sleep?' actually came from a dawning ability in father to do just that. The words in the dream show that father is *beginning to imagine himself* as being able to help his son. In a sense, therefore, a parent's dreams are one of the many aspects of caring for their children.

The baby in the room

What is the need for having the baby actually in the room? Sometimes there is a remarkable connection between what parents talk about and small babies' actions and vocalisations. Babies are often in tune with the emotional atmosphere and may cry when painful matters are being talked about. This can in fact be a clue to why some babies cry excessively; it may connect with some inconsolable experience in the parent's own history. When the parent is able to talk about this with the therapist, they may then be able to console the baby (Hopkins, 1994). The parent's reaction to a baby crying in the session may, in itself, be useful material for the work. Some mothers or fathers may deal with it by taking the baby out for a walk in the corridor, and it may seem to be an attempt to get away from painful issues stirred up in the room. Persuading the family to stay in the room can sometimes enable parents to share difficult feelings with each other for the first time.

With crying babies, mothers who have difficulty in soothing their babies may be trying to do so silently. When I pointed this out to one mother, she said, 'If I did say anything to him, it would be too horrible.' The opportunity to put into words to the therapist the 'horrible' thoughts that she had about the baby came as a release to her. Once such thoughts are said, and acknowledged, they may become bearable.

A therapist who is able to be non-judgemental can allow parents to own their hostile feelings towards the baby. In this case, it enabled the mother then to have a different range of feelings towards her baby. She became able to hold him close to her and to put into words what *he* might be feeling. She was no longer preoccupied with the force of her own impulses. The baby sensed this difference and was able to be comforted by his mother's holding of him. The therapist can be thought of as carrying out a symbolic holding of the emotions going around in a family; the experience of this holding enables parents to pass it on to their baby.

The therapeutic work must also deal with interactions that can be observed in the room. Parents may be helped to recognise babies' signals in a more varied way: at its simplest, this means that an approach by the baby to the mother may not always be for feeding; it may be for an interaction through speech or playing. In one family meeting about an eight-month-old who was being fed constantly, the father was holding the baby. When the baby started to grizzle, father started to hand him to mother. I asked, 'What would happen if you went on holding him?' Father said, 'He'll probably cry.' However, he did try holding on to the baby and was able to soothe him himself. Patterns of response can be thought about with an interested outsider, and altered.

Parent-infant work

I am here going to argue the importance of *parent*-infant rather than *mother*-infant work. Although most of us learned to work and think psychoanalytically with *individuals* in the first place, when we turned our attention to infants, we had to take account of Winnicott's saying, 'There is no such thing as a baby, only a baby and someone.' Walking on Hampstead Heath recently, I saw a stand-off between a father and a probably two-year-old boy. Each held their ground some distance apart so that the two-year-old looked as though he was on his own. Intrigued, I watched as every passer-by paused by the little boy and looked around until they spotted the father before moving on; interestingly, the ones most concerned were actually other children. In this incident, the 'someone' we all checked for was presumably the father. This 'someone' has until recently usually been thought of as the mother. It is time that fathers came in. It would be naïve today to assume that most babies are brought up in conventional two-parent families. But all babies needed a *father for their conception*. It is an essential part of knowing about any baby to know by what route their father comes to be either present or absent in their current lives.

Kenneth Wright (1991) talks of the vital role of the *father* in the structuring of the *self*, and the development of *symbols*; it is the mother who helps the first creation of structure in both the world and the infant's self. The father is initially in a third position, externally observing the mother-infant pair. A person in this third position guarantees the space for the child's thought and representation.

The Oedipus complex is one of the key discoveries of psychoanalysis, the one taken up most enthusiastically into common language. Ron Britton describes the Oedipal triangle very clearly (1991). He tells us how '[t]he closure of the Oedipal triangle by the recognition of the link joining the parents provides a limiting boundary for the internal world.' He calls this a triangular space. If this link between the parents, perceived in love and hate, can be tolerated in the child's mind, it allows a third position where the child is a *witness*, not a participant. If he can observe, he can also envisage *being* observed. This provides us with a capacity for seeing ourselves in interaction with others, for entertaining another point of view while retaining our own, for reflecting on ourselves while being ourselves (Britton, 1991: 86–7).

In a case of a *two*-parent family with a baby having very extreme sleep and separation problems, the problem was presented to me as being between mother and baby. The mother convincingly told me of problems with her own mother. I took in the seriousness of this but also wondered to myself about the relation *between the parents*. It seemed permissible for me to point out that the mother seemed to disqualify and discount the father's *different opinion* about the baby's needs, the theory of 'male insensitivity.' It seemed to me that I as the therapist/observer practised continence in not jumping in to become the potent third person to the mother-baby couple. Keeping in mind that the couple had a relationship that belonged to no one else, even if they were out of practice in it, seemed to help them back into it. The next meeting produced reports of changes between mother and baby that seemed to come from the *mother following the father's advice*. Perhaps also my ability to bear being the witness rather than the participant was reassuring to the baby as well as to its parents in the sessions. Babies often get more interested in the therapist when their parents become more interested in one another.

In this work, the need for careful listening to and observing of all the members of the family must be accompanied by similar listening to one's own countertransference. This countertransference must include *sympathy*, getting in tune with, and also *antipathy* to behaviour that is cruel or neglectful. The therapist must be able to *stand* not being in tune with aspects of behaviour even while understanding how this behaviour may have come about. This comprehensive stance may facilitate the parents not to split off their own judgement of their behaviour, and not to use projective identification to get professionals to have the only sense of what is a right way to treat a baby. Failure-to-thrive infants are one example where the danger of persecuted-feeling parents leaving the worry about the infant to professionals is *serious*.

In work with a family, transference and countertransference issues are multiple and complex. The therapist must judge, consciously or otherwise, *who* to attune to at any moment. We may at times feel attuned to where *both* parent and baby are. At other times there is real discordance. I was working with a depressed mother who cried as she talked. Looking at her, with a sympathetic expression, I then found myself looking at her baby, who was sitting with his face buried in her skirt. He looked up, caught my gaze and smiled at me broadly. I smiled in return. He was perhaps grateful for an adult who wasn't crying; he was probably also showing the means he may often have had resource to, a smile to cheer up his depressed mother. In any case I smiled back at him, then looked up again at his mother and was terribly conscious of my incongruent smile, feeling that I had to 'wipe the smile off my face.' It was a useful lesson for me of the dilemma for babies of depressed mothers – if their mothers cry will they make things better or worse by smiling?

Two embattled parents came with their sleepless baby. One (surprisingly in this case, the mother) told me that babies need firm boundaries. The father then told me that babies need to be responded to when they cried. A vista of boredom washed over me as I contemplated unpicking each of these assumptions.

With spontaneous impatience I said 'I think you're both right.' The parents seemed delighted and relieved, as though I had managed to contain their hostility and their conflicting opinions. It obliged them to discourse *with each other*, not just through me, and we could then all talk about how their own family experiences, where they had often felt put in the wrong, had led to their current beliefs about their baby.

Was my quip an enactment, a *failure* of attunement, or was it after all an ability to attune to the complexity of the situation? Both these parents were used to being told 'You're wrong!,' not just by each other in the present, but, as I discovered, by their unattuned parents in the past. Also, as we know, parents of crying babies often feel blamed by the baby. So my charming but rather sarcastic throwaway line may have had its use.

Another family I saw had an English father and a Chinese mother. Their ideas about child-rearing on first telling also sounded irreconcilable. But I noticed that, angry though they were, they sat comfortably in the room with one another, and both responded to their children. As the mother poured out her despair about 'laid-back English attitudes,' I said, 'you seem to be a one-woman campaign for Chinese discipline in Kentish Town.' Not a very subtle remark, but both parents laughed. Next week the mother told me that she felt the father had listened to her properly for the first time. They had been able to talk together at home. This empathy with both sides of irreconcilable feelings is a real art. You have to *not mind* what it feels like and not try too hard. Sometimes I think, 'Why do I have to listen to this?' as hatred spills out around me. At other times, I feel fortunate to be part of a living drama where I have helped emotions to be painfully expressed to some useful end.

Too much attunement can do families a disservice. Schlesinger (1994) points out that in conversation we often listen 'too closely' and lapse into identification with the speaker (quoted in Sternberg, 2002). When listening socially, we assume the speaker means to make sense and we fill in the elisions and ignore pauses, but this is useless in analysis. I similarly find when *observing* parent-infant interactions that, instead of *staying with noticing what is missing*, I may sometimes fill in the gaps in my own mind, and in a sense destroy the evidence of what is absent.

Colleagues Peter Toolan and Vivienne White recently told me of their reactions while seeing a three-year-old boy, Darren, and his family. Darren had serious behaviour difficulties, with a possible ADHD label. Peter reported having a 'splitting headache' after the session. During the meeting, Darren climbed up to reach something and hit his head on a cupboard really hard. His

> mother paid no attention to his injury. Darren became very subdued, clutching his head and burying himself into the seat. Vivienne suggested that he rub his head hard to take away the pain and he did this briefly. The mother commented that it was his own fault, that he never cries if he hurts himself and she made no attempt to go to him. A whole lifetime of interactive error is compressed into this brief statement. We see how each of the therapists enacts, or reacts, in a different way to this incident.

As a therapist similarly working with families with toddlers, I see many small accidents. These always arouse in me a feeling of a need for a certain sort of action. If this doesn't happen, I have a feeling of incompletion. When there is a fall or bump, it seems *essential* that the mother *touches* the injured part of the body as well as commenting on the injury. There must be a physiological imperative for this touching, as well as the emotional recognition of the hurt. What do we as therapists do when some essential action is missing? Vivienne was restrained in not rushing to soothe Darren herself, but she enabled him to soothe himself, perhaps a necessity for this boy.

A serious question that we all often ask ourselves: in the interests of not interfering, how much absence of what we feel is the right response can we *condone* on behalf of the child, or indeed *tolerate* on behalf of ourselves? Can providing some of what is missing show both child and parent that it does actually exist? – that heads that have been hurt can be rubbed better? Or must we address the underlying deficits in the parents' experience before interactional errors can be corrected? Indeed, do we show more respect to a parent by actually arguing from the evidence of what we have felt ourselves? Could Vivienne have clutched her *own* head, declaring to the mother, 'What a bang! Did *you* feel that?' Could she have said to Darren, 'Get your mummy to rub it better for you'?

Peter was as closely attuned to this incident as Vivienne was, but his reaction was different – he took a splitting headache away with him, presumably concretely in identification with the boy's pain as well as with the metaphorical pain of empathising with the struggles of this misattuned family. This example shows how two therapists working well together can absorb different aspects of a family's projections (and in fact as the work progressed, this family's attunement to their child's needs improved greatly). However, Beebe (Beebe and Lachmann, 2000) has noted that when mothers show non-attuned behaviour such as intrusiveness, their baby's heart rate goes up. Perhaps, even more frequently than Peter's headache, our blood pressure may be affected as a matter of course by getting in the way of these misdirected attunements! Kalin et al. (1995) have shown in primates that attachment behaviours operate on the brain of the mother as well as on the brain of the baby. How intimate need the contact be to have an effect? Perhaps even in a professional situation, therapists' brains are at risk from other people's disorganised attachments!

More optimistically, Regina Pally argues speculatively regarding psycho-analysis:

> Since it is known that consciously attending to and verbalising something can enhance cortical activation, it could theoretically be argued that treatments such as analysis enhance cortical functioning, and take advantage of its plasticity, to modulate deeply engrained emotional responses.
>
> (2000: 15)

Pally is writing about intensive psychoanalysis, but I suggest that in parent-infant psychotherapy where we touch, albeit briefly, on deep early processes, some major psychic changes also occur. I suspect that there must be equally an emotionally integrative effect for the therapist who goes through such a process with parents and their infants that is deeply satisfying. Ann Hurry has also recently written on this subject (1998: 54–7).

In this brief work 'character analysis' is not possible, but something truly characteristic in the way in which parents relate to their babies is got hold of. Serious listening to the problem as told by parents enables the therapist to think about *what* is told, *how* it is told, and what is *missing*. People who are properly listened to, and who are appreciated for who they are and what they have to face, may then be able to take on the ideas about themselves that start first in the therapist's mind. They may then start thinking for themselves, and perhaps creating some of what was missing.

Acknowledgement

Dilys Daws's work in primary care is funded by the Tavistock Institute of Medical Psychology.

Note

1 Maurice Whelan has recently edited a book, *Mistress of Her Own Thoughts (2000)*, which has brought Sharpe's work back into prominence.

References

Beebe, B., & Lachmann, F. M. (2000). *Infant Research and Adult Treatment. Co-Constructing Interactions*. Mahwah, NJ: Analytic Press.

Bion, W. R. (1962). 'A theory of thinking'. *International Journal of Psycho-Analysis*, 43: 306–14 (Reprinted in *Second Thoughts: Selected Papers on Psycho-Analysis*. New York: Jason Aronson, 1967, pp. 110–19).

Britton, R. (1991). 'The missing link: Parental sexuality in the Oedipus complex'. In: J. Steiner (Ed.), *The Oedipus Complex Today*. London: Karnac Books, pp. 86–7.

Daws, D. (1989). *Through the Night: Helping Parents and Sleepless Infants*. London: Free Association Books (Reprinted 1993).

Hartmann, E. (1973). *The Functions of Sleep*. New Haven, CT: Yale University Press.

Hopkins, J. (1994). 'Therapeutic intervention in infancy. Two contrasting cases of persistent crying'. *Psychoanalytic Psychotherapy*, 8: 141–52.

Hurry, A. (Ed.). (1998). *Psychoanalysis and Developmental Therapy*. London: Karnac Books.

Kalin, N. H., Shelton, S. E., & Lynn, D. E. (1995). 'Opiate systems in mother and infant primates coordinate intimate contact during reunion'. *Psychoneuroendocrinology*, 20: 735–42.

Kaplan-Solms, K., & Solms, M. (2000). *Clinical Studies in Neuro Psychoanalysis*. London: Karnac Books.

Main, M., Kaplan, N., & Cassidy, J. (1985). 'Security in infancy, childhood and adulthood: A move to the level of representation'. In: I. Bretherton & E. Waters (Eds.), *Growing Points of Attachment Theory and Research. Monographs of the Society for Research in Child Development*, 50 (29): 66–104.

Pally, R. (2000). *The Mind-Brain Relationship*. London: Karnac Books.

Palombo, S. (1978). *Dreaming and Memory*. New York: Basic Books.

Schlesinger, H. (1994). 'How the analyst listens: The pre-stages of interpretation'. *International Journal of Psycho-Analysis*, 75: 31–7.

Sharpe, E. (1940). 'Psycho-physical problems revealed in language: An examination of metaphor'. In: M. Brierley (Ed.), *Collected Papers on Psycho-Analysis*. London: Hogarth Press, 1978.

Sternberg, J. (2002). 'The relevance of the study of infant observation for becoming a psychoanalytic psychotherapist'. Unpublished PhD thesis. London: Tavistock Clinic.

Tronick, E. Z. (1989). 'Emotions and emotional communication in infants'. *American Psychologist*, 44 (2): 112–19.

Whelan, M. (Ed.). (2000). *Mistress of Her Own Thoughts: Ella Freeman Sharpe and the Practice of Psychoanalysis*. London: Rebus Press.

Winnicott, D. W. (1971). *Playing and Reality*. London: Tavistock.

Wright, K. (1991). *Vision and Separation between Mother and Baby*. Northvale, NJ: Jason Aronson.

5 Brief psychoanalytic therapy for sleep problems

Originally a chapter from **Parent-Infant Psychotherapy for Sleep Problems: Through the Night** *(2020), written with Sarah Sutton.*

Coming for help

My own work with infants who cannot sleep is in child health clinics, known as baby clinics, currently at a general medical practice and previously at the Tavistock Clinic, London. In both places, families bring problems with their babies' or small children's development. When families come with a sleep problem, it is always urgent and they need to be seen quickly. Although they may have been suffering with one or more sleepless children and apparently tolerating the situation for some time, when they do get to the point of seeking a referral, they often feel 'at the end of their tether' and bursting with emotion. They come in distress, in anger, overcome by helplessness. In looking at such problems with them, I have come to realise that the clue to the work lies within this emotionality. The strong feelings are not only the result of sleepless nights – they are also both a cause of the problem and a route into discovering how to alleviate it.

In spite of the urgency of the problem and often the distress of the entire family, I have found that as few as one or two consultations may allow a change in the parents' approach to the baby that breaks the deadlock between them. I usually find that if a change is going to occur, it does so after the first or second meeting; I then often see the family several times more to consolidate these changes. This is a departure from the longer-term intensive work of psychoanalytic child psychotherapy, and I will examine the principles underlying it.

It has been remarked that no one is ever the worse for having a sleep problem cured. What is more, sleeplessness, which can spread throughout a whole family, actually stops useful thinking by parents about what is going on in the family. Helping them think during the day can start a process that enables them

DOI: 10.4324/b23125-7

to manage the chaos of the night. When a sleep problem has been resolved, parents may deal more effectively with the normal run of the family's and children's developmental problems. However, curing a problem, without also having thought through its possible origins in the context of family relations, means at best that an opportunity for the family to look at their dynamics or their handling of their infant has been lost; at worst, the 'cure' may appear to confirm that the child alone was the problem.

Sleep disturbances often illustrate what is going on in a family, but families often need help to discover for themselves what is being represented by the problem. Also, issues uncovered between parents and children, or between the parents themselves, often lead back to parents' own experiences in their childhood with their parents. Repeatedly the theme of how to deal with and survive separations comes up.

Separation problems

Simplistically speaking, the problem for a mother in getting a baby to sleep is the basic act of putting the baby down, that is, of separating herself from her baby and the baby from her. McDougall (1974) describes how a baby needs to come to terms with the loss of the available mother and 'create psychic objects which will compensate for his loss.' His capacity to do this will be circumscribed by his parents' unconscious fears and desires. Through over-identification, many parents tend to spare their children 'the inevitable confrontation with reality. . . . The anxieties to which this primal separation give rise are usually qualified by terms such as annihilation and disintegration' (p. 438).

This conjures up for us powerful images of psychic processes. The consultations in which parents relate to me the details of their confused nights of wakings and feedings are a live illustration of the disintegration McDougall refers to. The fragmented experience which is conveyed to me starts to come together, as I listen to these details and make a more integrated pattern of them, initially within my own mind.

One extreme example illustrates this. The mother of Barnaby, aged four, and Clare, aged six months, had consulted many doctors and other professionals about many different complaints in herself and her children. She came in great distress about both children's sleeping problems. She talked non-stop about her many attempts to get help for this multitude of complaints and her confusion about what to attend to first. There was no dialogue between us, and ten minutes before the end of the session I stopped her to point out that she was leaving no time for *me* to talk. I then said that I had had two thoughts while she was talking. One was that it was very difficult to bring up children. The second was that she had consulted many professionals and that they had all got it wrong for her.

This mother was very taken by these thoughts. Because I offered no advice, I was in no danger of getting it wrong myself! More seriously, I had recognised that she was so full of conflicting anxieties that she had no space to let in yet another opinion. The next week, she brought her husband and both told me, very painfully, of their own difficult childhoods. I remarked that, as well as leaving them unsure of their individual ability as parents, their different childhood experiences had given them conflicting ideas of how to be parents; these were reinforced by contradictory ideas from the many professionals they had consulted.

Thinking about this enabled both to be more effective with their older child. Barnaby's alarming temper tantrums went within the next week and his sleep problems slightly improved. Their attention then turned to the baby, Clare, who was waking frequently during the night and needing to be breastfed by her mother. They repeatedly asked me, 'Should we leave her to cry?'

I described how there seemed to be no idea of any middle way between going to her every time and absolutely abandoning her. They then asked if it would make her feel insecure and damage her if she was left for a while. I said that perhaps we could turn the question around and think about how insecure it would make Clare feel if she thought that they *had* to come in to her every time she called out – that they could not trust her to manage for a while on her own and that they could not trust their love and care for her to carry on for a while from the last feed. The parents could feel, I think, that this reversal of mine was not superficial and 'gimmicky.' They could see I was moved by their accounts of their own childhood insecurity and the damage it had caused. While seriously keeping in mind the dangers of insecurity, I was able to suggest that Clare's position was not the same as theirs; with two loving parents safely at hand, *her* need was to experience herself as *separate* from them. They reported that when she cried they no longer went in, picked her up, and fed her. Each time she cried, they now would call out to her or go in and talk to her briefly, telling her to go to sleep. They said that her cries no longer sounded frantic, they were indignant or complaining or sad. Having thought about the meaning of Clare's cries, they then perceived the sound of them differently and were then also able to respond to them less frantically.

Barnaby and Clare's parents found the three or four consultations they had with me helpful; both children were happier and slept better. What made the difference? My choice of this family as the first clinical example in this chapter comes from two elements in the work: first, it was overwhelmingly evident that the parents' own childhood experience underlay their present problem in handling their children; second, they asked a question, 'Should we leave her to cry?,' that seemed to call irresistibly for a straight answer. In the response to such a question, we have the ideal chance to examine the differences and the common ground between this way of working and behaviour management colleagues who give more specific advice than I usually do.

Comparisons with behavioural work

Those who have well-structured programmes for parents to follow are of course also interested in and respectful of the relationships and situations of the families who consult them. But they may also be careful to define a cut-off point. For instance, Douglas and Richman suggest:

> In practice we have found that generally it is not useful to delve back into the past or into the parents' or the child's psyche to find out the cause of a sleep problem. It is more profitable to concentrate on the here and now of how parents are responding at night-time and how that might affect the sleep pattern.
>
> (1984: 47)

It seems from this that professionals may feel reticent about going too far into a family's privacy and that too much attention to the family's history is intrusive and not particularly relevant. I do not think this is quite right; in fact there is a deep human need to be known and understood. Sleep problems may often arise when families are having difficulty in straightforwardly under-standing and responding to each other. Even brief work where families are really listened to may enable them to feel that something crucial about them has been understood. They may then be better able to understand and respond to each other.

From informal comparisons, I gather that my own results in helping babies to sleep better, taken from the family's expressed satisfaction or otherwise, are similar to those of other workers. My impression, based on improvement claimed by families to have happened by the end of treatment, is that in half of all referrals there is a noticeable improvement in the baby's sleep. In looking at whether improvements last, and hold over the following year, for example, complications arise. Two opposing factors must be taken into account: first, that many sleep problems 'cure' themselves over time without treatment; sec-ond, that new stages of development in babies may lead to difficulties in sleep-ing. For any method of treatment, it is therefore worth considering how much 'success' at the time should be held to imply non-recurrence of the problem.

In comparing differing methods, it is interesting to speculate whether par-ents who are determined that they will solve the problem *now* can use whatever method is confidently offered or whether one method suits the personalities and needs of some families better. Several times I have seen parents who have previously had some behaviour management counselling and have then com-plained to me, 'They just told us what to do; they didn't *listen* to what *our* problem was'; but I suspect that as many parents have travelled in the opposite direction, complaining of me, 'She wouldn't give us any proper advice; she kept on asking us questions about ourselves.'

A psychotherapeutic method allows parents to work out for themselves important elements in their emotional relationship with their child. It seems that this might also help them deal with future problems. Behavioural work has equal, perhaps greater, success in alleviation of the problem, but less gain for the families in understanding for themselves the psychological pro-cess involved and in thinking about the origins of the disturbance. There are diagnostic implications here in assessing which families are able and willing to manage thinking about their family dynamics and which are not.

Here I must declare my debt to behaviour modifiers and the thought that they have put into the many questions that parents bring, such as, 'Should we leave her to cry?' Douglas and Richman (1984), for example, clarify different aspects of sleep problems and management techniques for solving them. Richman (1981a, 1981b) usefully differentiates between the causes of the sleep problem and the parental management which maintains it. Behavioural management addresses itself to this prolonging of a problem that no longer has a dynamic meaning for the child and its family. More recently, Ferber (2013) explores both problem and solution.

What most workers in this field have in common is struggling with the essence of the need a baby is expressing and communicating to his parents in waking and crying. What is less thought about is the way parents' hearing of their baby's crying is influenced by their own early experiences. Thus, 'Should you leave a baby to cry?' may initially mean, 'Should I have been left to cry?' The first consultation may in fact be a testing of how seriously the therapist, of whatever orientation, takes the 'cries' of the whole family for some understanding. The urgency of a baby's cries may stir up memories of similar infantile feelings of desperation in the parents themselves, which then render them incapable of acting as adult, competent parents. They identify with the baby's cries and are powerless to change them.

It is necessary then to look at the mixture of relief and hostility with which we ourselves, or the parents we work with, may greet advice which includes the concrete suggestion of leaving a baby to cry. The apparently simple question, 'Should you leave a baby to cry?,' contains parents' agonising and deeply felt doubts about whether their impulses are in fact cruel and sadistic. When their own desperate feelings have been thought about, they may also, like Clare's parents, hear the baby's cries as being less frantic.

Behaviour management techniques also deal with parents' fears by giving firm, sensible advice which tells them what is acceptable behaviour towards little children and what is not. In this way, it enables some parents to use common sense with their children. However, I think it is worth evaluating the logic behind these techniques. Among behaviour modifiers, there is considerable debate about different methods. Those who suggest letting a baby cry without picking him up may also emphasise the huge importance of checking on him and reassuring him of the parents' presence.

Weissbluth (1987) dismisses this checking as delaying the resolution of the problem and advocates leaving the baby alone until she falls asleep, citing many successful examples. His reasoning is that the baby quickly 'learns' to fall asleep and stay asleep and that the baby's ability to sleep in itself improves the relationship between parents and babies. However, in looking at this method we can see that it does not address the underlying relationship, although the change in the baby's behaviour may be a relief to all. Parents are switching from too much response to their baby to apparently none at all. Such an abrupt change of tactic could seem in itself as irrational as the previous practice. By contrast, in techniques where the parents remain near and responsive, the parents can be said to remain responsible to the baby for the change in their management of him. This takes some of the urgency out of the situation, as the baby's communication may be felt to be heard. The relief this entails may mean the baby goes on crying, or gives up and goes to sleep, but has been able to express his feelings to his parents about what is going on. Parents and baby are able to communicate and work something out between them.

Leach, in her book *Your Baby and Child* (2010), very clearly shows the dangers of simply leaving a baby to cry without going back to reassure him, explaining that if parents persist with this policy to a point where their child actually gives up crying, they have won the battle at a very high price. The child has been convinced that they did not care enough about him or understand him well enough to take any notice of what he was trying to communicate to them.

She considers the issue further in *Controlled Crying: What Parents Need to Know* (2015). Her advice is salutary, though it is also worth bearing in mind the ambivalent relationship which already exists between parents and children who have been listened to *too much* (Hopkins, 1996). Morrell and Steele (2003) suggest that when there are infants with a sensitive temperament, depressed mothers and ambivalent attachment, then 'the brief psychodynamic approach described by Daws (1989) may be particularly suited to parent-infant dyads with persistent sleeping problems.'

A parent's comparison of ways to solve the sleep problem

One mother of three little girls described to me her first baby's sleep problem at five months, two months after she had returned to work. Bridget refused to settle for the first stretch of sleep in the evening before her 11 o'clock feed. Her parents were desperate to have their own meal and do what was needed in the house, and her mother decided to use advice from a book which according to her said, 'Let them scream.' On the first night, Bridget screamed for three-quarters of an hour before falling asleep, on the second night for half an hour, and on the third night for only quarter of an hour. After two or three more nights of screaming for quarter of an hour, Bridget stopped screaming and settled quickly to sleep. Her mother, who had become exhausted, was relieved.

However, when the third daughter Anita also had a period of not being able to sleep, though at the later age of 12 months, her mother felt she needed very different attention. This little girl in fact used to get to sleep easily but later woke screaming. Her mother thought she suffered from nightmares and needed the reassurance and comfort of her mother's presence until she was able to fall asleep again in her cot.

It is interesting how differently this mother responded to these two babies' sleep disturbances. On the one hand, she was responding intuitively to different aspects of meaning in the wakefulness of the two babies. On the other, she also felt that her attitude to the younger child was coloured to some extent by what had happened between herself and the older one. Bridget's failure to go to sleep had indeed been cured very quickly, by leaving her to cry. Her mother was very thankful about this at the time. She could not have coped with more disturbed evenings. Nevertheless, she was left with an uneasy feeling of something unresolved between herself and Bridget, even though the 'cure' did not seem to have harmed Bridget. She was a secure little girl who coped very well with some later hospitalisation, when her mother stayed with her.

The transition for the mother from having a very wakeful baby, perhaps demanding attention because of her absence at work during the day, to having a baby who went to sleep quickly was gratifying, but it was also very abrupt. It is possible that what was missing for this mother in the few days of successful action was the chance to think through the implications for her relationship with Bridget of this enormous change. Perhaps the unfinished nature of this business with Bridget was what partly led to her different treatment of Anita, besides being the appropriate response to Anita at the time.

Reading baby books – the pitfalls

Reading books can be extremely helpful and supportive. St James-Roberts's (2012) book, *The Origins, Prevention and Treatment of Infant Crying and Sleeping Problems* is one such; a comprehensive guide to the many aspects of crying and sleeping that trouble babies and their parents. It summarises a wide range of research evidence and considers approaches to preventing or managing them. The limitation, though, for any book of guidance is that the parent/ reader cannot challenge their own questions as they bring them to the books in the way that a therapist can in an interview. The problem for parents in reading books giving advice about sleep problems is therefore whether the choice of advice to take fits in with and is reinforced by the kind of parenting they are already using or whether they are released to try something different.

For example, in a previous generation, Dr Benjamin Spock's (1946) advice to be sensitive to a child's needs came as a great relief to parents who had felt that earlier professional advice ignored the baby's own rhythms in favour of imposing an easily understood schedule of feeding and sleeping. When I chaired him giving a lecture to the Association of Child Psychotherapists in London in 1979, he was very complimentary about my success with sleep problems! However, Dr Spock's ideas could be interpreted by anti-authoritarian parents as a manifesto that any kind of discipline or limit setting was bad for children. Some of these parents may have been communicating their repudiation of the authoritarian style of their own parents. What they may not have been getting any more right than their parents was a sensitive discovery of what their baby's actual needs were.

More recently, behavioural approaches have been promoted purporting to offer tough love and no-nonsense rules, giving very specific advice to parents about behaviour-modifying schemes for getting children to sleep better, among other things. Programmes and books like this may rescue some parents from indecision and confusion, a feeling of not knowing what to do. The pitfall in such approaches, though, is that parents who are already insensitive to the meaning of their children's crying may use them as permission to go on ignoring the meaning. In our book for parents, *Finding Your Way with Your Baby* (Daws & de Rementeria, 2015), Alexandra de Rementeria and I hope to be open-minded. We say,

> This is the baby book that does not tell you what to do. We hope that it will encourage you to observe your baby, to really attend to the detail of what is happening in the moment and the feelings aroused in you. We are not 'teasing' you by withholding knowledge of what to do when there are problems. You know your own baby better than we can, and might be strengthened to find your own solutions. The book describes the emotions involved in having a baby and watching his development. In becoming a parent you develop too. Perhaps nothing else in your life changes you so much.
>
> (2015: 1)

One mother told her health visitor that her one-year-old baby slept about 12 hours at night but could not learn how to go back to sleep on his own if he woke. He woke once or twice a night and his mother used to go in, give him a bottle, and stay till he fell asleep again. She had now changed to giving him the bottle and a musical toy, instead of staying with him. She then announced a further change. She said, 'Today it's going to be a traumatic day,' because she would not give him the bottle any more. She would leave him just with the toy. She predicted that the baby would start screaming and she would come up after five minutes to stay with him. The next day she would come after ten minutes of crying. After a couple of weeks, he would get used to it and not need his mother or the bottle to help get him back to sleep. His mother then showed the health visitor the advice book she was using, looked through it, and said to the baby, 'You need a transitional object,' handing the baby several different soft toys. The baby wasn't interested and reached for his mother's book; she fetched him two of his own books instead.

In this account we see how a mother has decided to change the baby's behaviour without, apparently, any curiosity as to *why* the baby was still waking up in the night. At any rate, she did not pass on any such speculation to the health visitor. It may well be that, for whatever reason the baby was waking, both mother and baby were better served by an unbroken night's sleep, but even so one element would still be missing – the mother's *understanding* of the baby's waking, even while communicating that she was not prepared to tolerate it.

It was interesting that when this mother had an 'intellectual' idea that the baby needed a transitional object and artificially produced one, it did not work. However, she was sensitive to the baby showing her that the book she was using herself was important to him. She then brought the baby his own books. It may well be that the books did have a real transitional significance for the baby and, as something connected with his mother, were satisfying to him. This is what the essential nature of the transitional object, as described by Winnicott, involves; it has to do with an idea and memory of being with the mother that then enables the baby to be apart from the mother.

This moment of sensitivity by the mother highlights why she had felt that the day of withholding the bottle completely would be traumatic. The plan to remove the bottle from the baby, and hence remove the need for her to come in the night to supply it, seemed to be based *only* on the belief that the baby could/ should manage on his own. She was expressing no satisfaction at what she and the baby had achieved together in the mutual feeding relationship, nor was she expressing regret that she and the baby might be losing something between them. Moreover, there was no suggestion that the bottle itself might already have been partly a transitional object for the baby.

How parents use advice

Psychoanalytic work allows parents to put into words their conflicts about what to do and how to listen to the advice given to them. It may help them understand their fears of hostility and violence towards their children, by putting into words the feelings evoked by their baby crying. Paradoxically, it is sometimes those parents who seem most unable to set any limits who are most afraid that firmness might lead to cruelty. It is always vital to clarify what they are afraid of doing. Uninformed reassurance can be really dangerous. It can seem to troubled parents like a validation of their cruelty (which had not been recognised by the therapist) and might lead to them acting it out either passively, by leaving the baby for long periods, or actively, by physical means such as hitting or shaking.

Advice on bringing up children has always swung from one extreme to another, but no one is obliged to take it. It is therefore illuminating to look at the taking or ignoring of advice as an aspect of projection of the unwanted qualities of the self, such as cruelty. For example, getting a professional to recommend leaving a baby to cry is a way of getting someone else to take responsibility for worries about whether this is a cruel way of dealing with a baby. The parent is then free either to follow the advice without owning it or to repudiate it, attributing such advice to others and perhaps only looking at it in terms of cruelty and not, as in some contexts, useful firmness. In extreme cases, parents can project their own unacknowledged aggression so effectively that the professional's own aggression is stirred up and advice is given that does involve cruel or insensitive behaviour towards the baby.

Fraiberg's thoughts about parents looking at their own traumatic experiences are useful here: 'It is the parent who cannot remember his childhood feelings of pain and anxiety who will need to inflict his pain upon his child' (1980: 417). She describes how bringing back into conscious memory the *feelings* connected with experience, not just the experiences themselves, can break the chain of ill-treatment.

Whenever an apparently innocuous question by a parent is posed about whether to be more or less firm with a child, it is essential to think, 'Firmer than what?' In what context is the question being asked? Surprisingly often, some cruelty or neglect in the parents' own background is waiting to be revealed. But the telling of this is only the start. Is it the parents' hope that the therapist will condemn this cruelty, or collude with it and insist on repeating it, or dismiss it as irrelevant to present matters? All this has to be clarified. It need not be a lengthy business. These dilemmas have been carried around since childhood, but the therapist does not need to *solve* the problem for parents. Putting the present problem in its context may be enough to enable parents to go away and start thinking about it for themselves, possibly finding that other ways of dealing with the child have become open to them.

Taking these dilemmas one generation further, we see how children themselves, either as babies or later on in childhood, may have difficulty in knowing whether their parents have behaved cruelly to them. Hopkins (1986) describes how they have neither the experience nor the objectivity to evaluate their parents' behaviour towards them. It is difficult to discriminate between their own impulses towards their parents, their perception of their parents, and the real behaviour of the parents. It can take much effort in later life to sort this out.

The clinical setting

When working in a general practice baby clinic, referrals come to me from doctors, nurses, and health visitors. They may have known about the problem for some time and been working with it. Many such problems are in any case transitory; my colleagues usually consider a referral to me for some time, so as not to hand on the family prematurely. There may be a moment, with or without this background knowledge of the problem, when the professional realises that the family is desperate. Even so, when I am told about it, I do not usually feel that I should see the family immediately. I am, however, often able to see parents within a few days, and a gap of this length, knowing that they have an appointment, enables parents to think through the problem and perhaps come with a balance of vulnerability and defence, so that they can work with me as their adult parent selves, as well as convey to me some of their infantile desperation.

I do not ask parents to arrive the first time we meet with a written chart of their baby's sleeping and wakings. This could detract from the impact of the 'emotional evidence.' In behaviour management, making such charts can be a first stage in dealing with the chaos in the family. But I prefer to meet the family first in their state of chaos in order to be able to both feel and think about the implications of this state. However, it is then vital to start making a structure from the information they bring, though one that connects with emotions. As mentioned already, I do go through the details of what happens day and night with the baby and may take notes of such details in front of the family. Families may also wish to write things down between our meetings. These notes are sometimes the only way the family and I can remember, in later weeks, exactly how things were before and by what stages changes have been made. Otherwise, it can be hard to retain more than an impressionistic memory of the original situation.

Parents' use of the therapist

I do not usually comment on my use for parents in the sessions; I take for granted that I am doing a kind of parenting to them by my interested listening. Perhaps I am a combined parental figure, providing what could be described in a shorthand way as 'maternal' receptivity and 'paternal' limit setting. At other times, it does seem necessary for me to spell out what is happening between us. I am more likely to do this with sceptical and hostile parents, where I may point out how little expectation of help from me they seem to have. Sometimes, they will then link this to experiences with their own parents. With some parents, it seems necessary for anger to be experienced by parents and child towards me (and felt by me towards them) before anger can be comfortably dealt with in the family, and the parents freed to be ordinarily angry and firm with their child.

The length of treatment may be an important issue where parents use my support to take bold steps in separating from their child. They may wish me to remain with them, feeling they can manage new phases in their relationships only if this support remains. In work which is intended to be brief, this can indeed be a problem. One mother decided she no longer needed to take tranquillisers after I offered her some weekly sessions. This was a brave decision, but we needed to discuss whether the weekly times with me might become as addictive as she had feared the medication would be. Just as babies' use of their mothers, and vice versa, can be addictive, so there was a danger that this mother might need my continuing presence instead of being able to take away for herself the new ideas we had worked out together.

The nature of the problem can influence the parent's use of the therapist when, for example, there is an acute weaning problem and difficulty in separation. A mother's inability to say 'no' to her baby and her constant fitting in with his demands may be passed on as an expectation of how the therapist should behave towards mother and baby, that is, that she should fit in with them. One such mother was feeding her one-year-old baby constantly, night and day. She felt he could not stand it if his needs were not attended to at once. She herself was unusually specific about what times she could manage to see me and when she could not, although she was not working. I found myself feeling very unreasonable in not making special arrangements for her, until I saw these demands as a communication to me of what was going on between the baby and herself, that is, she was fitting in with his unreasonable demands as well as with his appropriate ones.

It will have become clear that I generally did this particular kind of work on my own, though in recent years I have changed this practice and enjoy the benefits of working with an experienced trainee. Working with a colleague changes the situation for both families and myself and has, as one might expect, both advantages and disadvantages. What is gained is another mind, another set of thoughts about a problem, someone who may see through one's blind spots. The co-worker can be a support to the therapist or help the family feel better looked after by a couple that is in some ways analogous to a parental couple. There are also losses. It can be harder for two people to pick up the unconscious links that are emerging from material. Simply by being different, a second person may pick up different, just as valid, themes, but in doing so may cut through the unfolding of something else. The delicate business of putting everything together in the therapist's mind is perhaps impaired by having two minds at work. One solution to these dilemmas is for the co-worker to be present mainly as an observer in the first meeting, joining in enough to prevent the awkwardness of being a totally silent presence, saying enough for the family to have a sense of who this person in the room is, but not cutting across the train of thought of the active therapist. This usually leads naturally on to the co-worker becoming active in later sessions. Such a method has great advantages for therapists training to do this kind of work.

The atmosphere of the consultations

Returning to thinking about individual work, consultations not only include a mass of information, but they are usually very lively. Babies cry; toddlers have to be taken to the lavatory, turn lights on and off, threaten to put their fingers in electric sockets. There is ample opportunity for families to show as well as describe how they deal with difficult situations. But what usually comes across is the parents' sense of freedom to use the occasion to look at this present problem of a baby who cannot sleep across barriers of painful memories of all kinds. Many mothers cry as they describe the birth of their baby and as they remember moments of pain, humiliation, relief, and joy. Sometimes I am shocked to find answering tears in my own eyes as I listen, but at the same time there is a moment of knowing that real emotion has been recollected and connected with the present. I have then been entrusted with knowing about the depth of feeling between parents and baby, however well or badly things might have gone.

If there is no flash of feeling, I am doubtful that anything will happen in the interview. One mother came, having recently taken her daughter into hospital, complaining that she could not cope with the baby's sleeplessness. The hospital had kept the baby a couple of days and sent her home again. This mother came to see me, looking worried and tense. She had no story to pour out and answered my questions dutifully, describing pregnancy and birth blankly. When I asked her about holding the baby for the first time, I again got a non-committal reply. When I said, 'Can you remember the first time she looked at you?,' the mother's face lit up in a smile. Suddenly she *was* remembering. This baby, who had become a worrying, persecuting problem, connected for a moment with the baby who had first looked at her mother at a few minutes old.

As with all infant-parent work, one of the main aims is to help parents see their babies more clearly, to look at them without misconceptions arising from misreading signals or re-creating old relationships.

Signals within the family

One essential factor is to pick up parents' feelings that I am being critical of them. This may come up in a reverse way, that is, *they* are critical of *my* way of looking at their problems. These feelings influence me when I wonder how much to tell parents of what I observe going on between them and their child in the room at the time. It can sometimes be useful to show parents ways in which they have got stuck in interpreting their children's signals, or it can be persecuting. It is sometimes hard to know beforehand how it will sound when put into words.

One mother came to me, complaining that her two-year-old daughter would not sleep and whined all day. She could not stand it any longer, she told me in an irritated moan. I took my courage in both hands and commented on her way of talking, adding that she and the child were looking at each other with equally disagreeable expressions. At the end of the hour I asked this mother, rather doubtfully, if she would like another appointment; she said she would and I anticipated another hour of moaning. But both came next week, bright and smiling, and the mother said how much better she felt. It seemed as though my remarks were experienced as a willingness to take on her disagreeableness. She started to tell me about her low opinion of herself and her capabilities. Over the next few weeks, she was able to get a part-time job and to start losing weight. As her self-esteem rose, she became more confident in her mothering; she and her daughter had happier times together and could sort out bedtime problems more freely.

Less successful was my attempt to show another mother whose child woke frequently in the night how I felt she misunderstood his signals. This 14-month-old little boy, John, fell as he explored my room. His mother swooped on him and picked him up with loud shrieks, before John himself had made any sound. John considered for a moment and responded by shrieking too. It seemed to me that John had neither been given time to work out his own reaction to his fall nor been comforted quietly. I thought it likely that something similar happened in the night, with John's mother reacting immediately to any sound or stirring from him, before really knowing if the sounds were a communication to her to come to him.

I commented to this mother on the sequence I had observed and realised I had offended her; the rest of the session did not go well. I told the health visitor of my tactlessness and she reported John's mother as saying that I had told her off. The health visitor advised her (and presumably me!) to give it another try. Next week during our meeting John fell again. His mother said nothing. John looked around in surprise, waited, and came to me for a response. His mother looked 'daggers' at me. I realised this was one family I was not going to be in tune with.

Equally daunting was Kevin's mother. She was a single mother with a two-year-old, Kevin; he had a one-year-old brother and she was again pregnant. Kevin woke frequently during the night. As they came into the room, Kevin jumped on a chair. His mother told him not to. I said I did not mind and his mother explained that if he jumped on the sofa at home, he could fall out of the window. I agreed that this was a serious matter and offered to fetch Kevin some more toys. His mother said, 'That's all right, he can jump on the furniture.' Kevin jumped and his mother said, 'Don't jump on the furniture.'

Surprisingly perhaps, this mother was quite happy for me to tell her how confusing I, and presumably Kevin, found this sequence. I connected it with what might be happening at night. With this 'double-bind' in force, Kevin would be very unsure of whether he was supposed to stay in his bed. Kevin came with his mother and little brother for several weeks; we played and talked together; his mother joined in and followed the children's play; and both children became able to concentrate better. Unhappily, this brief work was not enough; it did not last outside the room. Life at home was still chaotic, and Kevin's mother did not feel able to accept the offer of a place in a young family centre for long-term supportive work with her and the children.

What these last three families had in common was a misunderstanding or confusion about how to use signals among themselves and what to do with negative feelings about them. With the first family, my interest in them was enough to allow them to make pleasanter allowances for each other; in the second, the mother's misunderstanding of her son was compounded by her feeling that I also misunderstood *her*. In the third case, there was a feeling that I sympathetically understood the confusion, though this was unfortunately not enough to change anything.

The common element in my work with all three families was the attempt to enable the mother to observe the baby and her own responses to him. This can be supportive, when a mother is helped to see the meaning of her baby's cries and is gratified by discovering her own response to them. Some mothers even lack basic reassurance that their babies need and appreciate them. However, for some mothers it seems that the very acknowledgement of the baby's needs reinforces the problem. Mothers who have already felt alarmed by the life and death quality of an infant's basic needs, or by the strength of his emotional expression of them, will be additionally persecuted by having this pointed out. In such cases, the brief work described here may not be appropriate.

Secure adults are able to perceive their baby's signals; insecure ones may need to ignore them (Main et al., 1985). Being unwillingly made to perceive a baby's signals may thus interfere with the parents' defensive attempts not to look at issues of dependence, so very painful in their own backgrounds. An important consequence of looking at the meaning of behaviour between parents and baby during the meetings with me is that the parents also have the chance to start sorting out what goes on between themselves and their baby during the ordinary difficulties of the day. This can then carry over into a better understanding of each other during the nights, which can otherwise feel quite out of control.

Other workers confirm the value of some of the elements of the consultations I have been describing. One study of the relationship between sleep problems and other disturbances in family life reported, 'We had the impression that the interview itself was therapeutic for some mothers, as they reflected on their child's behaviour and family circumstances' (Lozoff et al., 1984: 182). Work with parents and child together brings out connections in their emotional states of being. These connections are also noted by Lebovici (1980), who takes account of what happens when the baby starts to cry during the session and suggests that perhaps some of the mother's own infantile feelings are expressed through her baby's cries. Often babies, apparently too young to understand the actual words, cry as parents talk about traumatic events in their own lives. I have noticed, for instance, that babies cry as parents talk about difficulties in their relationship. Following from this, we might think that at times a baby's crying in the night is connected with such feelings in the mother or, at any rate, that the mother's inability to comfort the crying baby comes from unresolved grief of her own.

The baby's physical setting at home

As well as looking at the complexities of the family relationships, the actual physical details of the problem, plus the parents' attempt to solve it, are considered in detail. Indeed one of the pleasures of the work is the problem-solving within a framework of physical objects and limitations – beds, cots, rooms, bath times – and the range of behaviours and activities that any set of parents feel is possible for them – lights on or off, doors open or closed, the availability of teddies, books, musical toys.

The way in which physical objects are described reflects the quality of the emotional relationships between parents and baby. If these are going reasonably well, parents treasure even their baby's clothes and blankets. Feelings about them spring from their feelings about the body they cover. Parents, of course, know minutely, and see meaning in, the baby's expressions and gestures, and they 'know' what is in their baby's mind. Following from this, the baby's toys are imbued for the parent with the meaning they have for the baby. I in turn picture all this vividly. Parenthood thus involves enjoying and being utterly involved with small objects and routinely performed actions. Similarly, it is necessary for me to have a mental involvement with the tiny details of what I am told about all this. Because I hear so many different versions, I am also aware of what is missing, of parents who are unable to create a routine or furnish their baby's environment with objects. I am then alerted to look at where this lack comes from, although I do not rush in to supply what is missing with my suggestions.

Methods of getting a baby to sleep

Barnaby and Clare's parents were fairly typical of parents who consult me when they told me how many different methods for handling their children they had used. They had tried so many ways, received so much advice, and none of it had worked. Moore and Ucko's (1957) study shows how variable handling seems to lead to a significantly higher proportion of chronically waking babies. They suggest a link between this and parental anxiety. The circular nature of this will be evident; cause and effect can get thoroughly blurred. Parents cannot always remember where they have started from to see whether something new makes a difference. One strength of behavioural technique is the way it can be helpful in sorting out the logic of making any change, in a way that parents can understand.

Another strength comes from looking at how one kind of behaviour by the baby links with another. For example, Paret (1983), in a study of waking and sleeping babies, shows that wakers could fall asleep only while being moved, held, or rocked. In one sample, 10 of the 11 babies in the waking groups could not be put down in their cribs until they were already asleep, whereas only one of the 19 good sleepers was rocked or moved to sleep (p. 174). Here we have some objective data showing that behaviour intended to help a baby sleep, that is, holding him until he falls asleep, does not also help him to stay asleep.

What difference does knowing this make to therapeutic work? I do in fact tell parents of this kind of connection and the conclusions it leads to. In particular, Ferber (2013) describes how a baby who falls asleep having been put into his cot awake then has the means to get himself to sleep again when he wakes up later. This is soundly based, logical information and is useful, both for its own sake and also in the context of looking at the assumptions behind methods parents have used that have proved unsuccessful, and their doubts and fears about trying other methods. These assumptions might involve the mother's ability to permit the baby to reduce his dependence on her and have other forms of gratification instead.

An important aspect of family consultations is of course the presence of the baby or small child themselves. This provides the invaluable opportunity to see how the members actually relate to each other. Not to be underestimated is the direct effect on the child of listening to the conversation. In fraught mother-baby relationships even quite a small baby can appear to respond to the therapist's attempts to 'hold' the mother and baby couple. It is easily apparent that older children are listening and making use of the issues discussed.

One three-year-old, who according to his parents had never been able to settle easily to sleep, said on the evening after the family's first visit to me, 'The lady said I have to go sleep,' and asked to be put to bed. It is touching that this little boy needed this simple 'instruction' so much that he had abstracted it from the conversation; I had not in fact directly addressed him in this way. What it allowed, in the following meetings, was a look at the dynamics of why the parents themselves had been unable to supply this much-needed, simple idea to their son and had had to seek my help.

The parents of another three-year-old boy, Noah, told me he had never slept well and had screamed for hours from the day he was brought home from hospital. His mother cried as she told me the details of his difficult birth and the fears she had had, first, that he would die and, second, that he was brain-damaged. Three times during the account Noah asked to go to the toilet and three times his father anxiously took him. On the second and third occasions, I commented on the fact that painful things were being talked about when Noah asked to go out. I was not meaning that he ought to stay in the room, but that his parents could start considering whether it would be helpful to Noah to hear his mother's fears about him openly stated. Meanwhile, we had the evidence that his father's first instinctive way of helping Noah in anxious situations was to allow him a change of scene, not try to hold him in one place. The immediacy of this, happening in the room, adds greatly to the picture of what happens at home at night when Noah cannot settle down to sleep. We see also in this family a vignette of one constellation of relationships. A vital aspect of the parental role is how much each is able to limit the other's misplaced concern about the child. This father, if anything, intensified the mother's concern, so there was no respite for Noah from his parents' anxieties.

One key factor in a sleep problem is the age of the baby when the family comes to seek help; the problem is very different with a three-month-old baby than it is with a three-year-old child. The issues of adjusting to the life and death demands of a very new baby are different from the negotiations with an older child. Richman (1981b) has pointed out that the origin of a problem and the forces that have maintained it as an ongoing conflict need to be disconnected.

Also of interest is the personality of the parents and their assumptions of what babies should be like. Raphael-Leff (1983, 1986) has made an interesting distinction between types of mothers she calls 'facilitators' and 'regulators.' In her view, regulators have more fixed ideas about how babies should fit in with their own lives and in fact have babies with fewer sleep problems; facilitators have more of an idea of fitting in with their babies and these babies have more sleep disturbances.

I have suggested here that a baby's sleep ability is coloured by the parents' own experience, as well as their perception of the whole question of sleeping, and I have proposed that experiences such as difficult births have a connection with sleep problems.

With most families, the presumed precipitating causes of the problem happened some time ago. What is often striking is that these families have already had a chance to talk over such events. Some seem to have forgotten that they have done so. What this suggests to me is that families who have had babies in intensive care or other traumatic experiences may need the chance to talk them through again at different moments in their baby's development. The continuance of a severe sleep or other emotional problem does not mean that talking through a difficult birth early on has not been helpful, but that it needs to be talked about again at different moments of the baby's continued survival and also needs to be talked about in the context of the parents' own childhood experience before it can be thoroughly dealt with.

One factor in perpetuating a family's apparent need for outside help may be that one vital element has not yet been taken up by any of the professionals prepared to listen. One such element may be anger with professionals for what has gone wrong at the birth or some other time. Furthermore, this anger may be displaced outside because of the parents' unbearable feeling of responsibility. A parent told me with scorn of all the advice doctors and health visitors had given her for her three-month-old son Patrick's acute colic. I said she did not seem to expect anything better from me. It took two or three meetings before I was able to show how she trapped unwary doctors into giving opinions she could 'prove' did not work. This made sense, as she saw how it connected with her feelings towards me. There may also be anger with parents' own parents for not being more supportive during a traumatic time. In the logic of the unconscious, if the parents feel responsible for the difficulties with their own baby, then *their* parents must be equally responsible for what has gone wrong for them. Such connections are not often put into words but continue as a reproach. Parents go on perpetuating a communication that someone has got it wrong, which wears out professionals. Finding the origin of this is an enormous relief to all concerned.

Working through it, in terms of feelings towards the therapist now, also allows change to happen. Most families I see do not really need more advice. They need to look at the process by which they have found it difficult to use the advice which is freely available. Either they have felt a conflict within themselves about what to do, or they have felt confused, not knowing which way to turn.

Where simple 'advice' from me does appear to be needed, we may be seeing unparented parents needing a grandmothering view to make up for a real lack. At other times, I suspect that when I am pressed to give advice, parents in conflict are trying to get me to support one parent's view against the other's, without having the conflict openly recognised.

Finally, a warning: sleep problems are usually a sign of concerned parents who are perhaps just rather confused in what they want for their child; sometimes, however, they can be danger signs of disturbed or very ill parents who are unable to be appropriately in tune with their baby's need to be looked after – they must then be taken very seriously.

References

Daws, D., & de Rementeria, A. (2015). *Finding Your Way With Your Baby: The Emotional Life of Parents and Babies*. London: Routledge.

Douglas, J., & Richman, N. (1984). *My Child Won't Sleep*. Harmondsworth: Penguin.

Ferber, R. (1987). 'The sleepless child'. In: C. Guilleminault (Ed.), *Sleep and Its Disorders in Children*. New York: Raven, pp. 141–63.

Ferber, R. (2013). *Solve Your Child's Sleep Problems*. London: Vermillion.

Fraiberg, S. H., et al. (1980). '"Ghosts in the nursery": A psychoanalytic approach to the problem of impaired infant-mother relationships'. In: S. H. Fraiberg (Ed.), *Clinical Studies in Infant Mental Health, the First Year of Life*. London: Tavistock Publications, p. 417.

Hopkins, J. (1986). 'Solving the mystery of monsters: Steps towards the recovery from trauma'. In: A. Horne & M. Lanyado (Eds.), *An Independent Mind: Collected Papers of Juliet Hopkins*. London: Routledge, 2015.

Hopkins, J. (1996). 'The dangers and deprivations of too-good mothering'. In: A. Horne & M. Lanyado (Eds.), *An Independent Mind: Collected Papers of Juliet Hopkins*. London: Routledge, 2015.

Leach, P. (2010). *Your Baby and Child*. London: Dorling Kindersley.

Leach, P. (2015). 'Controlled crying: What parents need to know'. *International Journal of Birth and Parent Education*, 2 (4): 13–17.

Lebovici, S. (1980). 'L'experience du psychoanalyste chez l'enfant et chez l'adulte devant le modèle de la nervosa infantile et de la nervosa de transfert'. *Revue Française de Psychoanalyse*, 44: 733–857.

Lozoff, B., et al. (1984). 'Co-sleeping in urban families with young children in the United States'. *Journal of Pediatrics*, 74: 171–82.

Main, M., et al. (1985). 'Security in infancy, childhood and adulthood: A move to the level of representation'. In: I. Bretherton & E. Waters (Eds.), *Growing Points of Attachment Theory and Research*. Monographs of the Society for Research in Child Development, vol. 50 (1–2, serial no. 209), pp. 66–104.

McDougall, J. (1974). 'The psychosoma and the psychoanalytic process'. *International Review of Psycho-Analysis*, 1: 437–59.

Moore, T., & Ucko, L. E. (1957). 'Night waking in early infancy'. *Archives of Disease in Early Childhood*, 32: 333–42.

Morrell, J., & Steele, H. (2003). 'The role of attachment security, temperament, maternal perception & care-giving behaviour in persistent infant sleeping problems'. *International Mental Health Journal*, 24 (5): 447–68.

Paret, I. (1983). 'Night waking and its relation to mother-infant interaction in nine-month-old infants'. In: J. D. Call, E. G. Galenson & R. L. Tyson (Eds.), *Frontiers of Infant Psychiatry*. New York: Basic, pp. 171–7.

Raphael-Leff, J. (1983). 'Facilitators and regulators: Two approaches to mothering'. *British Journal of Medical Psychology*, 56: 379–90.

Raphael-Leff, J. (1986). 'Facilitators and regulators: Conscious and unconscious processes in pregnancy and early motherhood'. *British Journal of Medical Psychology*, 59: 43–55.

Richman, N. (1981a). 'A community survey of characteristics of one- to two-year-olds with sleep disruptions'. *Journal of American Academy of Child Psychiatry*, 20: 281–91.

Richman, N. (1981b). 'Sleep problems in young children'. *Archives of Disease in Early Childhood*, 56: 491–3.

Spock, B. (1946). *Baby and Child Care*. New York: Pocket, 1957.

St. James-Roberts, I. (2012). *The Origins, Prevention and Treatment of Infant Crying and Sleeping Problems*. London: Routledge.

Weissbluth, M. (1987). *Sleep Well*. London: Unwin Paperbacks.

6 Feeding problems and relationship difficulties

Therapeutic work with parents and infants

Originally published in the Journal of Child Psychotherapy (1983, Vol. 9, No. 2).

Watching the behaviour of recently born lambs and their ewe mothers one Easter on a Welsh hillside, I saw the instinctive 'homing-in' by lambs to their mothers, and the searching and claiming by mothers of their offspring. Identifying at different times with one or the other, at one moment I was distressed when a lamb wandered bleating from one ewe to another, rebuffed by each one in turn: where was its mother? At other moments I felt myself flinching as lambs hurled themselves on their mothers and roughly and imperiously rooted straight onto their nipples.

It is obvious from these examples that something was going on about feeding as a part of a mother-infant relationship that aroused strong emotional reactions, even in an uninvolved outside observer. My first reactions were often of empathy with one or other of the nursing couple. I hope that as a devotee of parent-infant work, my ability to encompass both sides of the relationship was quickly mobilised. But it is relevant to point out that, in such an emotive area, any one of us can be drawn, without noticing it, to a one-sided view.

In this paper, I will look at infant feeding, both by breast and by bottle, in the context of the development of the relationship between the infant and its mother and father. I will not generally be thinking about the infant on his or her own, whether in the context of successful feeding, or of problems in feeding that would seem to stem from deep disturbances in the infant. Crucial is what the infant's parents bring to the relationship from their experience and memories of being with their own parents. Carrying on this theme all 'helpers,' such as doctors, nurses, or health visitors trying to assist in establishing feeding, or psychotherapists stepping in at a later stage, may have attributed to them some aspect of the ideas about parents that these mothers and fathers have in their minds.

DOI: 10.4324/b23125-8

The subject of infant feeding is so fraught because it is literally a matter of life and death: an infant not fed sufficiently and appropriately dies. Even if the result is not quite so stark, but things are going pretty badly, the result is 'failure to thrive.'

Parents thus factually have a responsibility to keep their baby alive – an awesome task. This calls on knowledge, skill, instinct, and emotionality. How does a new parent feel about being a parent, and about their new tiny helpless baby? Where do their emotions connect with instincts? How do love and hate fit into all this? One place where these matters are thought about is in the baby clinic of a general practice, where I work as a child psychotherapist one half day weekly. At a recent meeting, the practice members, general practitioners, health visitors, etc., went round in turn, each giving thumbnail sketches of the infants and young children that they knew of with feeding problems. The cumulative picture that emerged was that many of these infants' parents had an eating disorder themselves, and some also had evident personality or relationship problems. This impression is confirmed by Dahl and Sundeln (1986), who say that more parents of infants with feeding problems reported feeding difficulties in their own childhoods than would be expected by chance (quoted by Skuse & Wolke, 1992).

So in thinking about serious feeding problems, we are not concerned with simple technical problem-solving but with difficulties that already have a precedent, perhaps one could call it a history, in the family. Another way of describing it is that the feeding problem may be a symptom of a relationship problem. Of course with feeding, as with every other aspect of bringing up children, there are always difficulties, hesitations, panics about beginnings and endings, new situations to be thought about, experiments to be made. Heightened feelings about developmental stages are the ordinary dramas of family life.

However, in thinking about how an infant's feeding problem might connect with a similar problem in his or her parents, let us start with the mother's pregnancy. While not looking at this in depth, we can note that the mother's feelings about her own body and her emotional reaction to the pregnancy are going to be connected. Her feeling about feeding herself is going to colour her attitude to feeding the new life inside her. If she can nurture herself, she can also do it for the foetus. It is a crucial setting of the stage, that everything she concretely takes into her body, food, drink, medicines, etc., may have an effect on the baby and that every experience she has may in reality, or may feel to her in fantasy, affect the baby. Similarly, a mother who can breast-feed with ease may well feel in turn nurtured herself as she feeds the baby.

When the baby is born the mother continues to initiate and offer food, nourishment, and experience to the baby, but the enormous difference is that this now becomes an obviously two-person relationship, the first give and take. As Daniel Stern (1985) says, feeding is a somatic experience which 'requires the physical mediation of another.' Through feeding, a newborn baby and its mother start to get to know each other. The timing of the first feed is important, the sooner the better seems to be an important principle.

In their work on parent-infant bonding, Kennell et al. (1979) have shown how in the first hour after birth reciprocal interactions can take place between a mother, who is in a 'maternal sensitive period' at that time, and her baby, who is equally alert and active. During this time, the baby's eyes are wide open and he is even able to follow objects with his eyes and hands. After that he falls deeply asleep for three to four hours. Kennell et al. describe how in this early responsive period the initial stage towards parent-infant bonding can take place:

> We hypothesize that during this early sensitive period a series of reciprocal interactions begins between the mother and infant which bind them together and ensures the further development of attachment. The infant elicits behaviours from the mother which are satisfying to him, and the mother elicits behaviour from the infant that is rewarding to the mother. These interactions occur on many levels behavioural and physical. When the infant cries, his mother usually comes near and picks the baby up. The baby often quiets, opens his eyes, and will look at the mother and follow her with his eyes. During a feeding the mother may initiate the interaction. She may gently stroke the infant's cheek, eliciting the rooting reflex which brings his mouth in contact with his mother's nipple. Nursing is pleasurable to both the mother and infant, and it stimulates the secretion of oxytocin which causes the mother's uterus to rhythmically contract. . . . Because the maternal and infant behaviours complement each other the probability that interaction will occur is increased. These behaviours seem to be specific and programmed to initiate the process that bonds mother and infant in a sustained reciprocal rhythm.

As well as the emotional benefits, the immunities transferred to the child by the immuno-globulins and the T and B lymphocytes in the breast-milk give the infant increased protection against gastro-intestinal and respiratory infections. The infant is thus less likely to develop allergies, through this passive immunity. This immunising process gained through breast-feeding is of course critical for third world babies with their great vulnerability to diseases.

Winnicott (1947) describes the setting up of breast-feeding in poetic terms:

> Imagine a baby who has never had a feed. Hunger turns up, and the baby is ready to conceive of something; out of need the baby is ready to create a source of satisfaction, but there is no previous experience to show the baby what to expect. If at this moment the mother places her breast where the baby is ready to expect something, and if plenty of time is allowed for the infant to feel round, with mouth and hands, and perhaps with a sense of smell, the baby 'creates' just what is there to be found. The baby eventually gets the illusion that this real breast is exactly the thing that was created out of need, greed, and the first impulse of primitive loving. Sight, smell and taste register somewhere, and after a while the baby may

be creating something like the very breast that the mother has to offer. A thousand times before weaning the baby may be given just this particular introduction of external reality by one woman, the mother. A thousand times the feeling has existed that what was wanted was created, and found to be there. From this develops a belief that the world can contain what is wanted and needed, with the result that the baby has hope that there is a live relationship between inner reality and external reality, between innate primary creativity and the world at large which is shared by all.

Lest we get too carried away by the emotional powers of Winnicott's description we should, however, note a study reported in *The Lancet* (Cunningham et al., 1987), which showed that carrying a baby close had more effect on mother-infant attachment than the method of feeding by breast or bottle. Bottle feeding within a close physical and emotional context can be just as effective as breast-feeding for the future well-being and security of the baby.

It is interesting to speculate on the forces that lead mothers to feed by breast or by bottle. Joan Raphael-Leff (1991) vividly describes the personality constellations by which mothers could be described as 'facilitators' or 'regulators.' Facilitators (characteristically still in their dressing-gowns) include a majority of breast-feeding mothers; regulators are more likely to bottle-feed and more likely to stick to a time-table. Raphael-Leff points out that all mothers contain elements of both, and may be different with each of their babies.

Skuse and Wolke (1992) have noticed that breast-feeding mothers who keep to a strict time-table are also more likely to stop breast-feeding in the early weeks than mothers who feed on demand. Emotional factors may play a large part in this, but Skuse and Wolke point out that demand-fed babies are fed more often, and that 'frequent sucking stimulates the mother's secretion of prolactin which, in turn, contributes to an increased milk supply.' So demand does physiologically produce a supply which could make breast-feeding more satisfactory to mother and baby and lead to its easy continuance. It is important to remember that demand-feeding at this early stage is likely to be an accurate reading by the mother of the baby's signals that it needs to be fed. As the baby grows older, longer gaps between feeds become appropriate.

Feeding problems

What we think of as feeding problems divide fairly obviously into two main kinds, too much feeding, or too little. 'Too much' feeding usually means 'too often.' Although many different elements are contained in this, the dynamics are strikingly different from the 'too little' which usually includes a danger of 'failure to thrive.'

I will start first with the 'too much.' I am concerned here with babies in the early weeks and months. These are not the solid, overweight spoon-fed babies of the end of the first year. These are the younger, still mainly breast or bottle, milk-fed babies, who seem to be constantly having a suck at their mother's breast, or having a swig at yet another bottle. Where breast-feeding is concerned, physiological factors are important. Babies who do not have long enough feeds never get the high-calibre 'hind milk' which would really satisfy them. The 'hind-milk' after the baby has been sucking for some time is rich in protein and energy (Woolridge et al., 1980). Babies who suck very often but only briefly never elicit this nourishment and remain hungry.

Turning to emotional factors, little and often may mean that the mother is failing to read the baby's signals correctly; it does not always need a feed. It also means that there is no clear definition of when is a feed-time and when is not and there is no shape to the feed as an emotional encounter. From my interest originally in thinking about babies with severe sleep problems, it seemed that for many, the key problem was of separation between mother and baby. Some mothers were unable to put their baby down and be physically separate from them. Even with the current preference for keeping a baby close, carrying them during the day, sleeping with them at night, there still does seem to be a key factor of whether there is the ability not to be intrusive. This of course cuts both ways, a mother who can let her baby be; a baby who does not have to consume all the mother's attention.

Where there is little separation, underlying the apparent lack of respect of the other's privacy or individuality can, of course, lie deep-seated fear. Mothers who have to go on feeding their babies may seriously worry that if they do not immediately feed their baby each time it cries it will die of lack of nourishment. In one sense this is ludicrous, but in the presence of a mother and baby in the grip of this feeling, the logic seems inescapable. Mothers who endlessly feed their babies may also be expressing unending hunger in themselves and are not able to feel reciprocally fed and satisfied by their babies' satisfaction.

Therapeutic consultations

Let me now describe briefly the consultations in which I discuss these problems with parents. I always start by asking parents to tell me about the problem. I usually get a distressed account of how exhausted the parents, especially the mothers, feel about unremitting feeding. Of course, babies feeding constantly usually do so at the same rate through the night. Often the problem is referred as a sleep problem, but with the parents also feeling convinced that the baby wakes because it is hungry. The feeding problem and failure to get into a sleep pattern are therefore intertwined.

Ferber (1987) is severe about parents' misunderstanding of what the child's needs are and says they can actually cause or perpetuate the problem. 'Repeated feedings during the night only conditions the child to become hungry at these times. Therefore, it is likely that some of the extra wakings are actually triggered on this basis.'

Going back to the consultations, I then ask the parents about the baby's own history, about the pregnancy and birth, about the early weeks, especially about how feeding, breast or bottle, was established. I ask how the parents got together to start their relationship, and I ask about their own parenting, particularly what they know from their parents about their own early feeding. Often there is a small start of surprise as I ask this question. Some parents do have the family story about their own feeding firmly in their minds as part of the background to their practices with their own baby, others have not and are intrigued as they surmise a connection. There are things I have learned to look for as this story fits together: firstly the likelihood that the parents are having some difficulties between themselves, and secondly that the mother has mixed feelings about her own mother. Often when I ask what her mother is like I get an enthusiastic first reply, followed by some wistful remark about not seeing her often. It may be that ambivalences between a mother and daughter make for vulnerability in feeding a baby. The third factor ostensibly in the future, but immensely powerful in its effect on the present, is that the mother may be planning to go back to work.

As well as listening to this reported story, I also think about how some of this is communicated in the therapeutic consultation. I am aware of the principal ways in which I think the parents' attitude to me is a transference of aspects of the problems. Some mothers and fathers seem to experience me as an ideal mother figure who will understand them, listen to them and attend to their needs. Such parents may also try to extend the work with me. Families move into my room as though to spend an enjoyable hour basking in my attention. Anything I say is metabolised as soon as possible, my sharper remarks are acknowledged for their wit. They really enjoy me pointing out the family dynamics – but they do not intend to change. I am used to perpetuate the situation, not to help alter it. These, of course, are likely to be the families who idealise the feeding relationship. Others are very irritated by me and find me critical of them; everything I say is experienced as not quite right, as badly timed. They usually break off at a time that seems unexpected to me. I wonder about mistimings between themselves and the baby. (It reminds me of the milkmaid in Dylan Thomas's *Under Milk Wood* who was kissed when she wasn't looking but was never kissed again although she went on not looking!) In all these cases, pointing out the dynamics of their use of me, and of the structure of the consultations, can be useful. It may help parents think about similarities between this and how they get on with their baby, and indeed open up their ideas as to what they expect from, and how they deal with other important aspects of their lives.

Often parents will come describing very complex fraught feeding situations, and may then calm down with the experience of being listened to and taken seriously. Such parents tell their confused story as though expecting either an equally confused reaction, or the opposite, a very directive organising reaction. If they get neither of these, some will be disappointed and quickly go away, others will start to feel held by a steady thoughtfulness, and within this framework start to think for themselves.

An important concept in all of this is of ambivalence, that is to say unacknowledged ambivalence. Parents who can let themselves know of conflicting feelings of love and hate for their babies are in a much stronger position and may not need to act these feelings out so dramatically as those who do not know how to tolerate opposites. It often seems that mothers who let their babies feed constantly are not facing saying 'No' to the baby. It is as though feeding or being with the baby is seen as 'good,' spaces between as 'bad.' You could say that this leaves the baby without having had a feed with a definable beginning, middle, and end, followed by a time for digesting the food physically and the experience of the feed emotionally. It deprives the baby of the pleasures, both of memory and of anticipation. Moore and Ucko (1957) have interestingly pointed out that playtime after a feed is important in establishing sleep rhythms. Babies who spend 10 to 20 minutes in their mother's arms after they have finished sucking sleep better than those who spend either more or less time. It seems that mothers who offer this playtime are able to discriminate their baby's need for playful and loving contact with them, and do not confuse this with a need only for feeding. I also think that where the experience of the feed is unsatisfactory to both mother and baby, the temptation to keep going on to get it right may be strong. Difficulties in weaning may be a continuation of this process.

As well as thinking about what goes on between parents and baby, it is essential to try to understand what goes on inside each of them. Early feeding is about the reality of life and death; it is also about emotions that have a life and death force. Mothers have to face the impact of a baby's fears and greed and also deal with the infantile emotions stirred up in themselves by all this. A worker offering receptivity will equally be assailed by emotions coming from both baby and mother ranging from voracious greed to an inability to take in what is offered. Empathy with mother and baby can be exhausting and draining as though one is a demanding perplexed baby, or a mother who has no resources left, or exhilarated as though one is an ideal mother/grandmother who always has more to give. Any of these feelings need reflecting on; they may be a key to what either mother or baby feel they have, or what they feel they lack.

The dynamics of the 'failure to thrive' families are quite different from the constant feeders. I have seen fewer of these and will touch on it only briefly here. One obvious thought is that parents with a background of deprivation and neglect will feel they have little to give their babies. To describe it in even more dire terms, people who have really felt the food and sustenance they were given was begrudged them may have equally mean thoughts towards their own infants – they may never have had the chance to develop the altruism that allows people to share. One very worrying case I heard of recently concerned a mother who always made up less of a bottle-feed than she thought her very under-weight baby would take 'so as not to waste any.' Parents of 'failure to thrive' babies may sometimes apparently leave the worry to the professionals, who then feel themselves to be critical and persecuting of the parents when they express concern about the baby's progress or lack of it. A vicious circle of the parents feeling empty of any source of good feeding inside themselves and passing on the helplessness to professionals can continue. Under-feeding does not necessarily have the appearance of cruelty. Skuse and Wolke (1992) point out that 'breastfeeding may also lead to failure to thrive in the sense of poor weight gain, in a group of apparently contented yet chronically under-fed infants who give the impression of being satisfied after feeds.' They point out that these undemanding babies sleep for long periods and that they have 'mothers who do not respond to their infant's needs, but only to their demands.' Babies with a weak will to live, perhaps innate, may need more vitality than their parents can muster to pull them through.

First case example

Returning to the constant feeders, in one recent case a mother was referred to me because her five-month-old baby, George, was feeding two hourly night and day, and she was desperate. George had a two-year-old brother and the health visitor said that when he was a baby and had been breast-fed, she had never seen so much difficulty or panic in getting the feeding established.

I telephoned to arrange a time for the first meeting and suggested that the whole family come. Mother told me that 'the problem is just between me and the baby.' I acquiesced to this and offered a time the following week. When mother came into my room she looked round dismissively and said, 'It's rather dull isn't it.' I felt rather hurt on behalf of my serviceable NHS surroundings, and the Fra Angelico Annunciation which, by chance, is in that room. Mother then poured out a story of some desperate weeks in the life of this baby, of almost non-stop feedings, of the anguish of the two-year-old, of how her part-ner helped by taking over much of the care of the older child. I drew a blank in asking her to talk more about her partner at this point. She hurried on to tell me more about how difficult the children were. I asked about George's birth and she told me it had been relatively easy compared with the horrendous experi-ence with the first child. As she talked she looked much of the time at me; she fed the baby but did not look at him. I asked about her family, who seemed warm and very accessible. Her descriptions of her mother sounded genuinely supportive. No clues there as to why this young woman was so upset about feeding her baby.

We talked about his feeding – she feels when he cries that he must be hun-gry, so she feeds him. There seemed to be no space in her mind to think about why else he might cry. It emerged that she was bound shortly to go back to work – when she did she would have to have partly weaned the baby. I sug-gested that she was hanging on to feeding him so constantly because of a wish not to have to leave him. She retorted that she was longing to go back to work. She had a very high-powered job organising supplies. 'There's a war on, and I'm changing nappies.' I nastily said it sounded as though she felt the excite-ment was all outside the home and she naively agreed.

Mother seemed uneasy talking about relationships and in fact firmly said she wanted advice. She said she had tried to give the baby bottles, and so had his father to give her a rest, but he absolutely refused to take a bottle. I said perhaps a bottle felt to him like losing the breast, what seemed important was to help him manage for a longer time between feeds without anything. I suggested in the first place simply trying to change the habit of the feeds, and helping the baby last out for perhaps two and a quarter hours between each feed. Mother agreed to try this. It was time to go and she started to pack up hers and the baby's things. She turned the baby towards her, and for the first time (or at any rate the first time that I noticed) during the session, they both looked deeply at each other and smiled. She realised he had been a bit sick on the carpet and said, 'Well it isn't a precious Axminster,' but reluctantly mopped it up with a tissue. It took her quite a while to gather herself, baby, and possessions, and she left thanking me.

The following time she came in delighted that the feeds were stretched out a little longer. I was then able to get her to talk more about herself and her partner, pointing out that she had excluded him from our meetings. I increasingly got a barren picture of a family where little was done together. His family were close in themselves but she felt very excluded by their culture. She and her partner were not married, and she described how complex the wedding arrangements would have to be to suit both families. I said I felt she and her partner had not assimilated each other's backgrounds, the joint heritage they were passing on to their children. She said the local population was so mixed in culture that it was not an issue. Picking up her difficulty in focusing on her relationship with her partner, I asked baldly whether she thought she and her partner would spend the rest of their lives together, and she answered me seriously that she did not know. She was able then to talk more openly and honestly about their joint difficulties. She looked at and talked to the baby several times and kissed him during this meeting. She again left very lingeringly.

Next week, she rang and cancelled the meeting. She or the baby was ill. On the telephone I said how difficult the things we had talked about last time were. She denied this but accepted another appointment. She came the next week and told me of a further stretch of time between feeds – the baby was now going five hours in the night and I congratulated her on this. She then talked about the difficulty of managing both children. I said she was giving me a picture of two separate units, with the father looking after the older child and herself with the baby. I again suggested a family meeting and she said she did not want to get into this at the moment, she might later. She then said she was going back to work in a few weeks. It became clear that she was the main family breadwinner and was furious about her partner's failure to be so himself. I offered her a time the next week and (with my waiting list in mind) said that after that we might make the times fortnightly. Next week she cancelled, leaving a message that she did not need to come anymore. I rang back and spoke to her. She said she had now started back at work, had a good nanny, that the problems were solved because she was getting out. I said that I thought my changing the sessions to fortnightly had been a big shock to her. She said it had not made any difference and thanked me in a rather distant manner.

Discussion

With George and his mother, it seemed that two main issues had an influence on their relationship, namely the state of the parents' relationship and the mother's imminent return to work.

Firstly, the parents; when marriages go well the father can be one of the principal agents in getting a feeding relationship established. He can be protective, both as a bread-winner to allow mother time at home, and emotionally. Having provided this setting, some fathers may then feel jealous and excluded from the intimacy of breast-feeding, others can allow themselves to enjoy it vicariously. Fathers can also help mothers with 'limit setting' – they can represent the first stage of the pull of the outside world and hint at the excitement beyond the mother-infant duo. For this couple, it seemed as though they shared little. Many mothers with marital problems have a consoling relationship with their baby – perhaps being closer than the baby's own need would require. The ever-presence of the baby, who can get addicted to all this mothering, can then become very irritating to the mother. Mother's mother sounded warm and accessible, for many mothers the experience of this relationship could have been sufficiently protective and allowed her to flourish with her own babies; I wondered why it had not happened like this for George's mother. Had she been envious and felt excluded from her mother's relationship with her father? All this is speculation; I never got close enough to ask that sort of question.

Secondly, returning to work can very much affect the rhythm of breast-feeding. A separation, even though in the future, can spoil the feeling of timelessness which can be one of the enjoyments of a mother and infant's early weeks together. A separation that is because of the mother going back to work can also lead to her failing to take responsibility for it herself – the job will be taking her away, not her own wish to be separate at times. This can make it difficult for her to create and own very small separations between herself and the baby in the present, such as simply the space between feeds. This in turn has a critical effect on setting up sleep patterns; babies get used to waking up repeatedly to feed (Daws, 1989).

In summing up the work with George and his mother, it is essential to note that the problem she came with, of cutting down the feeds, was greatly improved. I was left feeling dissatisfied because I had been allowed a glimpse of so many relationship issues, without then having the chance to discuss them properly. It would seem that this difficulty in going into things emotional would be a characteristic of how she was with important people in her life, not just with me in these sessions. She lingered with me and found it very hard to leave, but then cancelled a session, and really chopped off the end of the work. I was both led on into involvement and then prematurely dismissed. How much the change to fortnightly meetings was disturbing to her I do not know. She knew that this was brief work, but perhaps some past major separation was stirred up for her. It must also be considered whether my cutting down her time was partly a retaliation by me for her cancellations, or an identification by me with her 'desertion' of the baby by going back to work. Whatever they were, I do think that the emotions I experienced with her must also have been felt by others, especially her baby, and her husband. It was tantalising that we never got to talk about this.

Second case

A second family came with a baby, Anne, aged four months, with very similar sleep and constant feeding problems. This family, in contrast, were only too keen to talk about their problems. Mother experienced the birth as horrific, in a hospital she disliked, because she had intended to have a home birth. She had a caesarean and woke to find Anne on her breast. Mother was really worried that Anne had suffered from the manner of her birth. Because she had planned to have the baby at home, she had not chosen the hospital and said that she got the worst one possible. They did not remove all the placenta and ten days later whilst alone with Anne she haemorrhaged and 'stupidly,' she said, went back to the same hospital and had a D & C. I asked why she had so much wanted a home delivery and she said she hated hospitals.

I asked both parents about their own families. The parents, from different incompatible backgrounds, had met in London. Both had travelled a great distance, partly to get away from difficult families. Mother was the middle one of five children and her father had died three years ago. I asked if her mother had seen the baby and was told that she had visited early on. Mother had not wanted her to come, but father had persuaded her to invite grandmother. Mother said she does not get on with her, though it had been good letting her see Anne. Father said, 'You hate her. You said you wished she was dead.' Mother looked abashed. I said I thought it might be difficult having had a girl baby if things were like that between her and her mother. Mother agreed, half laughing.

Father also told of a problematic family who could not talk about emotions, with parents who kept secrets from the children. He was now a banker, and mother told me of despising money, of hating living in the suburbs, and of getting sucked back into the middle class. She was also very lonely and did not know how to find congenial friends.

I said I was starting to see a pattern in the way mother hated structured hospitals, banks, the middle classes, and that I wondered if there was a clue to the problem between her and Anne, i.e. it was difficult for her to help Anne get into a structure of more time between feeds, and that she was not giving Anne a chance to learn anything about structures and how to adapt herself to them. Mother, agreeing, said, 'I'm teaching her to be just like me.'

We talked more about the details of Anne's feeding – she goes to sleep from the breast, though mother tries to catch a moment to put her down just before she really is asleep. Anne will not suck a dummy, but they are seeing if she will take bottles with expressed milk. She does not suck her thumb but does manage to suck her fist. They thought she could in fact settle herself to sleep when she wakes at night, but mother herself sleeps badly and springs awake when Anne does. During the day mother takes her out, and at weekends both parents go for long walks with Anne in a sling. While they keep moving, she does not need to be fed. Father said they have tried solid foods; it does not seem to stop her needing frequent feeds, but perhaps they have not done this for long enough yet.

During this meeting, I commented several times on Anne's responsive smiling at her parents. She played with some bright wooden beads and put them in her mouth. At times she also smiled at me. I said she did not seem like a discontented baby, and I thought she needed help with lasting out longer between feeds. It seemed as though all the emotional issues in the family were affecting her, but we could also see whether the practical steps of trying to change the pattern of the daytime feeds could help change the constant feeding at night.

With this family, we see how they were able to use me and seemed relieved to talk openly of emotional issues. In later sessions, I was able to look much more directly at interactions between mother and Anne and to use my own feelings as part of my observations.

In one such meeting, Anne cried. Mother tried, with my encouragement, to delay feeding her. Anne's cries became more distraught. Mother clutched her, stood up, and paced the room with Anne on her shoulder. I pointed out to mother that she was silent, not saying anything to Anne. (I have often noticed that mothers who are unable to console their babies are silent while they cry.) Mother was amazed, she had never thought of this. She started to talk to Anne, but by now it seemed to be too late. Anne's crying was so urgent that I also felt that only feeding would do. The feeling pervaded the room so strongly that I actually found myself saying to the parents that I felt as though I needed to be fed. This rather bizarre remark of mine did not seem to disconcert them. My countertransference empathic thought gave me a clue as to why it was so difficult for them not to feed her at once – her cries perhaps resounded with their own desperate, and I think unanswered, cries to their families. Although the only solution at the moment in the session seemed to be to feed Anne, mother did start to talk more to Anne at home. In fact, as their communication by such means grew, it became less necessary for Anne's mouth on mother's nipple to be their main form of contact. As frequently happens to babies in this situation, Anne started to babble and to use her mouth and hands much more for play.

Discussion

It seemed as though my ability to put feelings into words were what helped this family to look at, and start to manage, some of their own emotions. This mother and father both felt unsupported by their own parents and had started their marriage in a spirit of opposition to all that their parents represented. However, they were able to use me, even though one of the 'establishment' in an NHS clinic. They were, perhaps, hungry for some confirmation of themselves as parents from a 'parent-figure' and enjoyed my interest in them. My response to them, by identifying with each of them, with Anne and the strength of her infantile needs, and with the parents' despair at satisfying her, made them feel that someone understood. In such cases, parents mobilise more resources, and the baby, sensing this, may become less distraught.

It does seem that a fixed response to a baby's crying of always feeding may actually be a failure to understand the communication in the crying.

Recently I said goodbye to a family with a 15-month-old boy that I had worked with. When Robert and his parents first came, at seven months. he fed night and day and screamed much of the time in between. This time they came to the room with Robert walking confidently, smiling with recognition at my toys and naming them as he played with them. He got mildly upset at one moment and father said to him relaxedly, 'I don't understand what the problem is.' Robert was satisfied with father's response and pointed out something about a toy car.

Parents (like Anne's) in the grip of a pre-verbal infant's anguished crying may not be able to give their baby the comforting message that they are trying to understand.

Conclusion

Early infant feeding problems can often be understood through the relationship between parents and their infant. Feeding difficulties later on may be a continuation of these problems, or they may be new issues stirred up by weaning and the feelings connected with losing the breast or bottle and the first intimate relationship that these imply. The psychotherapist's counter-transference, the feelings evoked as she listens and observes, is an important tool in understanding and 'feeding back' to the family what she has discovered. If the parents can take this in, a process of change between themselves and the baby may then take place.

References

Cunningham, N., Anisfeld, E., Casper, V., & Nozyce, M. (1987). 'Infant carrying, breast-feeding and mother-infant relations'. *The Lancet* (February 14): 379.

Dahl, M., & Sundeln, C. (1986). 'Early feeding problems in an affluent society (i) determinants'. *Acta Paediatrica Scandinavica*, 75: 380–7.

Daws, D. (1989). *Through the Night: Helping Parents and Sleepless Infants*. London: Free Association Books (Now updated, 2020).

Ferber, R. (1987). 'The sleepless child'. In: C. Guilleminault (Ed.), *Sleep and Its Disorders in Children*. New York: Raven, pp. 141–63.

Kennell, J. A., Voos, D. K., & Klaus, M. A. H. (1979). 'Parent-infant bonding'. In: J. Osofsky (Ed.), *Handbook of Infant Development*. New York: Wiley, pp. 786–98.

Moore, T., & Ucko, L. E. (1957). 'Night waking in early infancy'. *Archives of Disease in Early Childhood*, 32: 333–42.

Raphael-Leff, J. (1991). *Psychological Processes of Childbearing*. London: Chapman and Hall.

Skuse, D., & Wolke, D. (1992). 'The nature and consequences of feeding problems in infancy'. In: P. J. Cooper & A. Sten (Eds.), *Feeding Problems and Eating Disorders in Children and Adolescents, Monographs in Clinical Pediatrics, 5*. Philadelphia: Harwood Academic Publishers.

Stern, D. (1985). *The Interpersonal World of the Infant*. New York: Basic Books.

Thomas, D. (1954). *Under Milk Wood*. London: Dent, 1991.

Winnicott, D. W. (1947). 'Further thoughts on babies as persons'. In: *The Child, the Family, and the Outside World*. Harmondsworth: Penguin, 1964.

Woolridge, M. W., Baum, J. D., & Drewett, R. F. (1980). 'Does a change in the composition of human milk offset sucking pattens and milk intake?' *The Lancet*, 2: 1292–4.

7   The perils of intimacy

Closeness and distance in feeding and weaning

Originally published in the Journal of Child Psychotherapy (1997, Vol. 23, No. 2).

Thoughts about the feeding of infants include an idea of both closeness and distance between two people (Parker, 1993). In work on eating disorders in young people, the intrusiveness, or its opposite, the unavailability, of objects is often described. The experience of this may have been internalised in infancy.

In an earlier paper, I wrote about how feeding is established and how weaning develops (Daws, 1993). Problems discussed were mainly about babies who were fed 'too much' or 'too often' and I describe this as a separation problem. Parents and babies could manage closeness but could not work out how to pull apart. Bereavements or other losses often seem to underlie this problem in separating; equally important is ambivalence or unacknowledged hostility in the mother.

I look now at the opposite, babies who seem to be fed too little, and may in extreme examples 'fail to thrive.' One way of describing their situation is in the *distance* between their caretaker and themselves. Worries about such babies are very often first noticed and reported by health visitors, pragmatically in the form of concern about *the way the baby is held for a feed.* It would of course be simplistic to think of physical closeness as 'good' and distance as being a 'bad thing.' The regulating of distance may be a crucial way of managing emotional issues. In other words, an avoidant attachment may, for some mothers and babies, be the best they can do in their dealings with each other. Juliet Hopkins (1996) has shown that the 'too good' mother, who follows the baby too closely, may not allow space for development.

In a quick look through some of the papers about failure to thrive, I saw how this dialectic between distance and closeness is mirrored, with the usual polarity of a race through the wide literature versus the closer single case study. It is difficult to change pace from one to another, and, for instance, in a useful annotation on 'The Process of Parenting in Failure to Thrive,' Boddy and

DOI: 10.4324/b23125-9

Skuse (1994) are clearly irritated by Shapiro et al.'s (1980) argument that 'it is the mother who is the key' in failure to thrive, on the basis, as Boddy and Skuse complain, of the clinical evaluation of a single family.

Yet most of us clinicians gain our inspiration from our 'single cases.' Perhaps we idealise and over-generalise what we learn. We do, of course, all walk around as personal single-case studies; our own early feeding whether remembered, cold to us or not, may be the underpinning of our approach to the topic now. In fact, as a researcher, David Skuse, like Alan Stein and colleagues, illustrates brilliantly in his video-studies the personal experiences, the pleasures, and miseries of particular parent-infant feeding couples.

By taking part in and teaching infant observation (Miller et al., 1989), we have invaluable individual examples of mothers and infants getting the feeding relationship going. I quote from an observation of a baby at three and a half weeks. In what seems like a very normal, pleasant situation, you can see how high the level of anxiety is, how it is put into words and, with luck, processed. The observer writes:

> The baby did not appear to be stirring. Mother goes on to say that R. continues to be very hungry, wanting to be fed every two hours or so. I ask about the night time. Together mother and father explain that initially R's cot was at the foot of their bed and they had swapped their pillows round to the foot of the bed so as to be nearer her. Mother had had to prod her every now and again because she was so still while she slept. Now they had the courage to move their pillows back and be a bit further away. She starts out the night in her cot after having a bottle. During the night after a feed she joins them in the bed, and is there handy for breast-feeding next time she wakes. Mother and father were amazed that they didn't squash her, though mother commented that her sleep was very different and that she heard the slightest noise from the baby.
>
> Father commented that sometimes no cause could be found for her crying. Mother said she felt that she did recognise some of her cries. Every now and again she seemed to be in complete agony and you could see her face crease up and her legs pull up. They thought it was colic. The doctor had reassured them, although he did not know exactly what the problem might be. They had looked up colic in the books and were horrified to find that colic went on for *only* three or four months.
>
> R. had begun to stir, moving her head and screwing her face up. Mother said that she felt that babies' cries were designed to make you pick them up and that she thought people who said you should let them cry a bit before you pick them up were wrong.
>
> R. began to cry quite gently and mother went over to her and picked her up and said hello to her. Mother asks her if she should get her bosoms out for her. She does so and R. takes a minute or so to latch on and begin sucking.

Mother is attentive to R. but carries on talking. She says it's difficult to know how much she's getting, that breast feeding has been rather a struggle. She's persisting but is still having to give her bottles as well, though she knows she needs to cut them out as soon as she can. She rang a Breast-feeding Advice Line during the week who said, 'Everyone can breastfeed, my daughter is still breastfeeding her two-year old'. Mother felt that they did not offer any really constructive advice.

R. *is* still being fed. She screws her face up and begins to go red, very suddenly she starts to wail. Mother sits her up, talks to her and jigs her, she calms down and mother asks me if I would like to hold her while she gets ready to give her the other breast. I take her from mother and sit her on my leg. My hands seem much too big for her, I sit her on my leg, though it would be easier to hold her against my body, at my shoulder. She begins to cry again and mother is ready now so I pass her back saying something about her knowing what she wants. This time she latches on immediately and seems to be sucking with enthusiasm. Unfortunately, it's time for me to go.

In this account, you can see how absorbed both mother and father are with the idea of just where to be in relation to their baby. They are able to experiment with different constellations of breast, or bottle, and move their pillows around as confidence comes and goes. The observer is also sensitive to ideas of physical distance, she helpfully holds the baby when asked to by the mother, notes the baby's size in relation to her own, and says, 'I sit her on my leg, though it would be easier to hold her against my body, at my shoulder.' She is torn between two very strong feelings, one an instinct that babies need to be held close and beyond it that babies stir up feelings of wanting to hold them close. On the other hand, she feels that in the presence of a baby's parents this would be over-intimate. This matter of fact aside by the observer about a very personal reaction gives us a vital diagnostic clue in our thoughts about closeness and distance between a baby and its caretakers. Closeness seems to be an essential ingredient; when it is absent we need to think about what the distance represents. In this vein, a second example of an infant observation with a baby three weeks old:

She then started dressing M, the crying started and soon became very strenuous. Her little face became very contorted and bright red. Mother picked M up and held her against her chest and the crying immediately stopped. This happened two more times, mother asked if she was going to have to feed a half-dressed baby? At that stage, mother seemed to have made the decision that M was going to have to scream until she was finished dressing her. During this time, mother was laughing rather nervously and said, 'Oh, you are horrible – you have no patience at all'. When the dressing was completed, mother picked up the baby and held her close, saying, 'Now you are probably going to eat my scarf'. The crying ceased, but M had put part of her fist into her mouth and was sucking away.

Mother then sat in a chair and placed M. on her lap and positioned a tissue under M.'s chin. I was aware of thinking how very neat and tidy and almost perfect everything seemed to have to be.

M was held close to mother and eagerly took the teat of the bottle and mother made some remark about her greediness again. Throughout the feed, M's gaze was centred on mother's face. Her left hand had been brought up to the bottle and even though her fingers were not around it, there was a sense of her holding onto the bottle. Mother commented that 'Soon she'll be holding the bottle herself.'

I think the account of this feed is painful to listen to and especially this last remark 'soon she will be holding the bottle herself.' We see how mother's interpretation of the baby's holding is seen as the first steps towards independence. If the baby had been breastfed and had stroked the mother's breast while feeding, this would more likely have been seen as a sign of the baby's closeness, of a wish to hold on to the mother (I will come later to an example from a baby I observed many years ago).

At six weeks, the observer was distressed to see the mother hold the baby on her lap in a fairly upright position, with space between her own body and the baby's:

Mother supported the back of the baby's head in her left hand, an arm's length away and fed the baby the bottle with her right hand. I was aware of feeling uncomfortable about this positioning of the baby for the feed, wanting mother to place her against her own body for a closer, more intimate position. The baby seemed only interested in the bottle rather than her position and eagerly started sucking away.

However, later mother does settle the baby back into a closer, more intimate position against her own body, with her arm around the baby. When the baby was 18 weeks old, we see her well into the swing of solid foods, eaten from a little high chair. This was followed by a bottle held by mother and the observer noting, 'In total there must have been a distance of about two feet between mother and baby (the distance of mother's outstretched arm).'

In thinking about this baby whom mother describes as 'greedy' and 'a little monster,' it is important to remember that she *is* well-fed. She is not failing to thrive. This mother had to manage times of her husband being away on business. We could only guess at whether the space between her and her baby that seemed so painfully wide to the observer is a representation of this gap, or of others in the mother's experience. Additionally, we might think that this way of putting a distance between them is her way of *managing* the complexities of intimacy. Would closeness be even worse?

It is important to think of where a mother's direction of experience is in her distancing from the baby. Is it paranoid or depressive? This mother seems to be anticipating damage to herself from the baby's greed, symbolised by 'Now you are probably going to eat my scarf.' Another mother might be protective of the child. One mother, referred to me *with* her baby, never looked at him, never caught his gaze. By holding both of them within my own gaze, I tried to release the possibility of her looking at him. Then, more actively, I looked at the baby myself, smiled and talked to him, pointing out his (somewhat bleak) responsive gaze. I found myself needing to say that I was noticing that she did not look at him. Mother said, 'I'm afraid I will damage him,' a surprisingly articulated comment within the context of this non-contact. She meanwhile told me a story of her own isolation and of her hatred of the baby's father. In one sense, it was impressive that she wanted to protect her baby from this, but the route she had chosen may turn out to be a chilling life sentence for him.

I turn now to Juliet Hopkins's description of helping a foster-mother to respect the distance that a child she is caring for *needs* as the preferred space between them (1994). In this case, Hannah, aged six months, was referred to her by a paediatrician for persistent crying and not making eye contact. She had been born to a single schizophrenic mother and moved to the foster home at one month. The warm-hearted foster-mother, Martha, told Hopkins 'It's worse than crying, it's piercing screams.' When the baby woke with a startle:

> Martha lifted her gently onto her lap while talking kindly to her and showed me how Hannah sat stiffly, not moulding to Martha's body. Most striking to observe, Hannah held her legs raised above Martha's lap and Martha explained that Hannah never let her legs rest on Martha's body. Hannah had already rejected cuddling and Martha showed me how Hannah strained away from her chest when she drew towards her. She told me that holding her when she screamed made her cry more.

She also told Hopkins that Hannah had drunk more milk from a propped bottle in hospital than she did on Martha's lap.

In this one session, Hopkins and the foster-mother built up a picture of Hannah as a baby different from Martha's own children: a nervous supersensitive baby who had a bad start in life, who felt overwhelmed and frightened by people when exposed to face, voice, and physical contact all together but who dearly enjoyed relationships with her family when they were modulated:

> Martha was pleased that I felt it would be all right to continue with the propped bottle, to leave Hannah alone in her cot and not try to cuddle her when she resisted. She thought she would buy her a rocking chair. I was aware I had given her permission to take her cues from the baby. After this one session only, Hannah made eye contact with the foster mother and her husband that same day, became more smiley and friendly and screamed

less. Hannah could not make eye contact until Martha saw her need for distance through more accepting eyes.

Paradoxically, it was Juliet Hopkins's brilliant ability to make a meaningful emotional contact with the foster-mother that allowed her to be more restrained in her approaches to Hannah.

In contrast to baby M, whose mother interpreted her holding on to the bottle as a sign of being ready to manage by herself, I now give an example of the baby I observed over 30 years ago. This was in fact one of the babies quoted by Esther Bick in her paper on infant observation (1964). The observation began when baby James was four and a half weeks old. The quotation goes:

When mother put him on to the breast he attached himself to the nipple at once and sucked vigorously. He had his eyes open and with the right hand he touched the breast and the button on the mother's dress alternately. This touching of the mother's body was observed as a regular pattern of behaviour whenever the baby came close to her. At thirteen weeks, the mother gave the observer the baby to hold while she went out to prepare the bath and said, 'Go to your auntie, she's got to study you'. James lay on the observer's lap looking at her, but did not touch her. When the mother returned he looked at her and followed her with his eyes until she took him. On her lap he felt for the breast with mouth and hand and later held her arm with his hand. After the bath, at the breast, he clutched at the breast; his mother removed his hand. He then put his hand on top of the mother's hand and moved it rhythmically while he sucked. At twenty-two weeks he was stroking the breast with wide movements. 'At twenty-four weeks' (I am quoting from the student's notes) 'James took the breast eagerly. His mother said he would not be having it much longer, the milk was giving out. With his left hand James played with the mother's breast and then with her hand. His movements remained lively all through the taking of the breast. As I watched him I wondered if his movements might be a conscious caressing of the mother; he appeared to me to be aware of what his hand was doing. The mother put James to the second breast and he took this eagerly, stroking her breast and neck and touching her mouth. He was weaned to the bottle at twenty-seven weeks. There followed a week of distress when he refused food, falling asleep between mouthfuls, whilst sleeping badly at night. The mother remarked that he behaved as though he was a little baby. In the following week he started touching the bottle, later reaching out for it, stroking it lovingly, as he had done with the breast, and eventually settled down to keeping one hand on the bottle and touching, stroking, and caressing the mother with the other hand.

We see in this how the baby James lovingly unites the experiences of the breast and the bottle.

Breast or bottle

Again we can see how the choice of breast or bottle may be a function of how the mother perceives the distance between herself and her baby. Let me say here that feeding a baby is a life and death issue: babies die if not properly fed. It is also about emotions that have a life and death force. Some mothers always intend to bottle-feed; breast-feeding feels to be out of the question. Others may breast-feed happily, while yet others start to breast-feed but have to give up. Some of these may be overwhelmed by failure, others feel that the bottle rescues them from something unmanageable, and they can harness their resources much more successfully with the bottle as a sort of mediator between them and the baby. Winnicott (1968), however, said that the survival of the mother was more of a miracle in breast-feeding than in bottle-feeding, an implication that something is missed in bottle-feeding.

One mother I worked with had tried to breast-feed but had difficulties from the start. Going away with her husband to stay with his mother, she struggled on and made several fraught telephone calls to the health visitor. The health visitor, at a distance, felt helpless and mother moved the baby onto a bottle. They came home and things settled down and the health visitor paid special attention to her, knowing that this mother's own mother had died when she was six months old. There was obviously a great deal to talk about and the health visitor referred mother and baby to me when he was five weeks old. I then had a chance to hear the upsetting story of the mother's wish to breast-feed her baby and how it had seemed to go wrong. She was able to tell me about her mother's death and her memories of a very miserable childhood, which included other losses. I said I thought she had not been able to breast-feed her baby because she wanted to spare him *her* experience of being intimate with her mother and then having a sudden total loss. Nothing could be worse than that. The mother found this thought of mine enlightening. She was then able to allow herself to see how close she actually was to her bottle-fed baby, who was large, smiling, and delightful. She next brought her husband to meet me and they did further work together on the resentments left by both their difficult childhoods, which perhaps helped consolidate their fairly new relationship with each other.

Failure to thrive

Perhaps the most famous example of a failure-to-thrive baby in the psychoanalytic literature is Shapiro, Fraiberg, and Adelson's study (1980) of Billy, referred at five months in a 'grave nutritional state, the baby was starving,' in one of the most stark accounts any of us will have heard:

> Then Billy uttered sounds of complaint. His mother said that it was time for his bottle and volunteered to feed Billy. She said 'Watch what he does when I show him the bottle'. She placed the bottle on the floor several feet away from Billy, who was on hands and knees. Billy's face

registered alertness and urgency – no smile, but urgency. And the 5 month old baby began to creep the long distance towards the bottle. He reached for it unsteadily but could not quite grasp it at first. Finally he did grasp it, mouth open hungrily, but it was bottom up. He could not quite orient it. At last he got the nipple into his mouth. He sucked solemnly, greedily.

While I watched this scene, masking my own inner pain and horror, the school girl mother explained that this was the way Billy took his bottle. 'He likes it that way. He likes to have his bottle alone, on the floor.'

Shapiro continues that it soon became clear that neither Kathy nor the father had any real sense of how much food Billy needed. Actual hunger was part of their daily experience, and they had to limit their own appetites severely in many ways. At some level, both Kathy and John seemed to feel that Billy would *simply have to share in their hunger*. Apparently, they did not fully understand that his life was at risk.

As the therapist worked with the mother on her own isolation and need to be mothered, her ability to respond to Billy improved:

When Kathy's own cries were heard by me, she began to respond to her baby's cries. When Kathy's needs were understood by me, she began to interpret the signs of needs in her baby. When hostile feelings towards Billy could be put into words, they no longer exerted their influence in distancing Kathy from Billy, she was free to enjoy him. When the powerful ambivalence towards her own mother came into the therapeutic work, Kathy completed her own adolescence and became free of the 'witch-mother' who impeded her own development as wife and mother.

This last paragraph also encapsulates the philosophy of parent-infant psychotherapy as we have learnt it from Selma Fraiberg. The idea that we need to listen to the parents' cries before they can hear their babies' cries is crucial. In another paper, 'Ghosts in the Nursery' (1980), she equally powerfully shows how some parents are unable to recognise their babies' needs because of their own unmet needs. I think this sums up in a nutshell the situation where babies are simply not given enough food. Their parents do not notice their need, or cannot respond to it, or feel they have no resources to give the baby, or do not wish to share the resources they have. To the professionals, seeing an underweight, neglected baby, the cruelty in the parental attitude is apparent. In one very distressing case I heard about recently, a newborn baby was removed from his mother at three weeks, after gaining no weight at all since birth. He had an older sister a year old and it occurred to the workers that, in order to deal with her jealousy, she had been allowed to displace the baby, being given first place at the breast. The baby's needs had not been thought about. However, the little girl was also not really provided for. During a meeting with the mother she indicated that she was hungry. Mother vaguely said she had a banana for her but could not find it. Not till the end of the meeting did she find it in her coat pocket. Such instances are rightly unbearable. Hanging on to Fraiberg's belief that attention to the parent is essential to help them mobilise something for the baby can be very difficult in such cases. At times, it may be inappropriate to persist, and care for the baby elsewhere may be unavoidable.

Similarly, in a clear and useful paper, Ruth Selwyn (1993) describes failure to thrive as 'associated with the impairment of the mother's capacity to nourish her infant, both in the material and psychological sense.' She says, 'It seems that our listening and helping mother to make sense of her experiences and feelings was felt by her to be nurturing and supporting. Noticing her needs and getting to know her helped her to be more available to her baby.'

Feeding and attachment

Poor feeders

It is necessary to look at attachment issues to understand why, when food is ostensibly freely available, some children are unable to take it. Skuse (1993) notices that '[c]hildren who are persistently poor feeders just do not seem to be as motivated by appetite as the rest of us.' Later he says, 'It is important to be aware that infants who fail to thrive at the breast comprise two fairly distinct groups. Firstly are those who are restless, who cry excessively, who may not complete their feeds or who latch on inadequately to the nipple.' We can see that, in Bion's terms, these may be infants who do not feel sufficiently contained by the mother. There are of course physiological explanations for some infants' difficulties in learning how to feed. Here, however, we are looking at the emotional components of such problems. The difficulties as listed by Skuse could well turn into the sort of behaviour which is currently described as Attention Deficit Disorder. Where better to look at its causation than at the breast? In Skuse's second and, as he says, less well-recognised group are infants who appear to have little appetite, do not demand to be fed and so may go excessively long periods between feeds. He says:

> Growth failure may occur as a consequence of a far more subtle interaction between infant characteristics and parental response. In a recent whole population survey of infants who were failing to thrive within a disadvantaged inner city area, we found that about two out of three infants tended to 'sleep through feeds' (whether breast or bottle, before or after weaning) at some point in the first post-natal year. The great majority, 80% of mothers in a well growing comparison group, regularly woke their children on these occasions, but only 50% of mothers of failing to thrive babies said they did so.

A recent article by Dieter Wolke (1996) is simplistic in arguing about the interpretation of such material. He believes it shows that maternal deprivation is not the cause of underfeeding other than in a small minority of cases. I think he is missing a subtle interaction in which we might hazard that depression in mother and/or infant plays a part. Similarly, Pinheiro (1993) argues, from six selected case studies, that 'infants' problems in taking food would correspond to difficulties in processing emotional experience, as expressed by the parents, and in the parent-infant relationship.' It also takes us back to Shapiro's patient, Billy, whose parents felt that he would have to share in their hunger.

Famine conditions

To widen the argument, Antoine Guedeney (1995) has pointed out that, in famine conditions, whether babies survive or not may relate to attachments. He suggests that infant depression, related to uprooted families who have lost home and family members, in turn leads to a lower survival rate. Where food is in short supply for everyone, survival depends in part on the quality of relationships that help to keep people going.

Weaning

Weaning from the breast can feel like a traumatic loss to mother and baby or like a time of achievement. How this goes may relate partly to the role of the father in the family. If what he brings is seen as support for mother and baby in the first place, and then leading in to newness and excitement and also limit-setting, perhaps this paves the way for weaning. If father is marginalised, felt to get in the way of an idealised mother-baby duo, then weaning might seem to be a disaster. Difficulties in weaning may highlight unresolved problems in the feeding relationship and problems with breast or bottle can continue into the offering of solid food to a baby. One mother at this point desperately said that she always knew she would have a baby with feeding problems.

Weaning is the long process that includes the introduction of solid foods, the lessening, and finally giving up of breast-feeding or of bottlefeeding. It is now recommended that babies start solid foods at 16 weeks or so. A baby taking solid foods can be pictured as held by mother or as sitting up in a specially supporting chair, graduating to sitting up independently in a high chair. The spoon is a new element, something that does not have the direct connection of mouth and nipple or mouth and bottle teat. The spoon, held by the mother and going into the baby's mouth, can be seen by each of them. We have a new partnership, mother and baby getting together about a third thing. And anyone can join in. Weaned babies can be fed by father, grandmother, and the whole family. Eating solid foods is a whole new skill and Skuse and Wolke (1992a) vividly describe the whole process of opening the mouth, chewing, swallowing, etc.

> In the early days of spoon feeding the food may be scraped off the spoon into the mouth with the lower jaw and tongue acting in concert. The tongue may protrude as the jaw opens, almost as if it is anticipating

suckling food. However, eventually the normal infant is able to inhibit tongue movement in anticipation of food reaching the mouth. In order to swallow efficiently it is absolutely necessary for the tip of the tongue to be carefully controlled. It is elevated and pressed up against the hard palate. Good tongue control is essential for the efficient ingestion of non-fluids. As infants move from the nipple to the spoon or cup new coordination patterns must be developed. The initial rhythm for the emerging sequence is not well established, but eventually the development of smoother rhythm patterns give a mature appearance to sucking, swallowing, chewing.

The earliest chewing pattern is often described as 'munching'. It is similar in rhythm to early suckling and seems to evolve from the combined patterns of suckling and biting behaviours. As chewing matures, the jaw, tongue and lip behavioural patterns become integrated into a smooth rhythm with flowing movements. The first consistency of food that is usually given is very soft and can essentially melt under the action of saliva. Munching seems to develop from the combination of two primitive patterns, the phasic bite reflex and sucking.

(Evans-Morris, 1977)

Connected with all this is the emergence of teeth. In the later part of the first year, babies may delight in their teeth, in their hardness, and in the ability to bite. Biting may express newly recognised aggressive feelings. Teeth also means having to be careful about biting – perhaps the essence of reaching the depressive position is having to feel sorry about biting your mother's breast. Being able to bite into hard biscuits takes the worry out of getting your teeth into something and weaning may be a relief. However, following one of our lines of thought about babies who are not thriving, perhaps depression subdues the biting impulses, and some babies may have a poor appetite because of this.

These physiological developments are a delight to most parents. To others, they are a source of serious worry, even to the point of a phobic anxiety. I have, for example, recently seen a family convinced that their baby was unable to chew and swallow solid food, in a way that seemed to link with a difficulty in getting hold of aggressive currents in life generally for this family. How this pervading atmosphere got translated into a specific symptom in the baby is one of the fascinations of psychosomatic functioning. From my recent reading, it occurs to me that the particular expertise of a speech therapist, making the connections between mouth and throat feel less of a dangerous mystery, might have been helpful to this family. We should also take note that speech delays and feeding difficulties often go together.

Sitting up is an important stage in child development. It coincides broadly with the detachment and changed emotionality that Klein described as the depressive position. We can also picture a sitting-up baby being able to get efficiently into the rhythm of spoon-feeding with another person with 'turn-taking' as a part of this. There is also the essence of looking with some-one else at a third thing. The breast-feeding infant's narrow focus, with two eyes on her mother's eyes, changes to the wider span of the older baby sit-ting up on mother's lap with four eyes turned to look at the same object. In Mary Cassatt's marvellous paintings, mother's and child's bodies are together occupied in a moment that looks infinite. Daniel Stern (1985) picks up the sense of this in his unpoetically named RIGS – repeated interactions that are generalised. He says,

> The generalized episode is not a specific memory. It does not describe an event that actually ever happened exactly that way. It contains multiple specific memories, but as a structure it is closer to an abstract representa-tion, as that term is used clinically.

We can see thus in Cassatt's painting of The Bath an abstraction of the close-ness of many bath-times. Similarly, the experience of a feed is abstracted from many different events. It is one of the underpinnings of psychoanalytic think-ing that the repeated reliable events of early feeding allow intimacy to develop and the experience of trust in others.

At this stage, a baby who is being weaned already feels somewhat separate from his mother. The weaning is built on a loss that has already happened. Weaning is about new experiences, including different combinations of bottle, spoon, and feeding cup. It allows for new tastes and new feelings about these. The spoon can represent a continuation of mother; it also leads into the baby's opportunity to feed himself, in identification with his mother, and also instead of his mother. Trevarthan and Hubley (1978) describe a stage of 'secondary intersubjectivity' at about nine months when the baby is interested in people and also objects, and in the situation between the two. The baby recognises the mental life of the mother, including her skills, and becomes interested in copy-ing her and learning from her. At that point, the baby can learn how to use tools, including the spoon.

In a popular leaflet for mothers from the Health Education Council, 'Start-ing your baby on solid foods,' pictures of spoons charged *with* suitable foods, illustrate the advice given. Prominent also are pictures of babies whose mouths seem to claim our attention. I would like to turn here to the feeding difficulties brilliantly illustrated by Alan Stein et al. (1994) and in other studies by David Skuse (Skuse & Wolke, 1992b). They refer to videos with actual moments, captured on the camera, and probably representative of many others. In Alan Stein et al.'s painful scenes of mothers unsuccessfully spoon-feeding their one-year-olds the spoon seems either to come intrusively at the wrong moment or, alternatively, is offered so tentatively or nebulously that it does not seem to be there to be got hold of. David Skuse has recorded equally frustrating scenes of small children restlessly roaming around their home, not seeming to be anchored by a feeding person.

In the ordinary wisdom of advice to mothers (Health Education Author-ity, 1995), we are told of the connection between infants' and parents' problems.

> It may be that your child is picking up your own feelings about food. Perhaps you're a dieter or have a weight problem, or maybe you just see healthy eating as a very important goal. If your child is picking up on your anxiety it may be that mealtimes have become an ideal time to get attention.
> Just as anxiety may cause problems with toilet training, it can also cre-ate problems with eating. So try and take a step back and think about how much of a problem there really is.

Eating disorders and feeding difficulties

Alan Stein et al. (1994) look at mothers with eating disorders to see what feeding difficulties they had with their children. They found there was evi-dence for 'an association between the presence of maternal eating disorder psychopathology and impaired quality of mother-infant interaction and infant growth.' Mothers with an eating disorder were more intrusive and critical than the controls during both mealtimes and play. They missed their babies' cues and were less able to set aside their own concerns. They showed more conflict with their infants during mealtimes, especially about mess and about who held the spoon, and their infants were less cheerful during both mealtimes and play. The infants of mothers concerned about their own shape tended to be lighter than those of the controls. However, some of the mothers with eating disorders did interact well with their children.

Play and feeding

The connecting of play and feeding fits in with the finding I have quoted elsewhere (Daws, 1993) from Moore and Ucko (1957) that play at the breast of a certain length is a predictor of good sleep. Babies who spent 10–20 min-utes in their mother's arms after they had finished sucking, slept better than those who spent either more or less time. It seems that mothers who offer this moderate amount of playtime are able to discriminate their baby's need for playful and loving contact with them and do not confuse this with the need for feeding.

On this theme, Pollitt et al. (1978), in a prospective study, considered whether mother and infant behaviour during feeding would predict infant growth during the first month of life. They carried out standardised ratings of maternal and infant behaviour during feeding interaction when the child was 20–36 hours old and noted that children whose mothers switched to a non-feeding activity during the feed (for example, cleaning the infant) gained less weight. We see here how inappropriate behaviour by the mother destroys the continuity of the feeding. Such mothers perhaps produce some of the restless behaviour at the breast that I quoted earlier from Skuse. In thinking about the process going on when mothers are, as Stein says, 'intrusive,' we are helped by some thoughts from Christopher Bollas. He has coined the term 'extractive introjection.' He says:

> I believe there is a process that can be as destructive as projective identi-fication in its violation of the spirit of mutual relating. Indeed, I am think-ing of an intersubjective procedure that is almost exactly its reverse, a process that I propose to call **extractive introjection.** Extractive introjec-tion occurs when one person steals for a certain period of time (from a few seconds or minutes, to a lifetime) an element of another individual's psychic life.
>
> (Bollas, 1987: 158)

He further describes this in relation to play.

> **B** is a four-year-old at play. . . . the parent enters the scene and appropri-ates the playing by telling the child what the play is about and then pre-maturely engages in playfulness. **B** might continue to play, but a sense of spontaneity would diminish and be replaced by expectant gameful-ness. If every time **B** is spontaneously playful the mother or father takes over the play and embellishes it with their own 'play', the child will come to experience an extraction of that element of himself: his **capac-ity** to play.
>
> (Bollas, 1987: 159)

Stein et al. cite the parents who are intrusive both at play and in a feeding situ-ation. Briggs (1997) calls this kind of feeding 'an injection.' We can see how a small child intruded on in this way may feel that the capacity to imagine tak-ing in the food has been spoilt. The parent has taken away the meaning of the toys in play or the spoon in feeding so that the child can act only through the parent's volition. Winnicott's transitional space (1971) has been obliterated. In play, Winnicott says, the 'Baby's view of the object *is* subjective and the mother is oriented towards the making actual of what the baby is ready to find.' We can think of the spoon as having the characteristics of a transitional object and think that it represents a link with the mother and at the same time a mov-ing away from her.

In Winnicott's summary of the qualities of the transitional object, the first is 'The infant assumes rights over the object and we agree to this assumption.' It would seem from this that the infant needs to assume and be given rights over the spoon in order to be able to feed himself. In the famous spatula paper, Winnicott (1941) describes the way in which a baby manages to get hold of and take possession of an attractive shiny object. In the first stage, 'The baby puts his hand to the spatula but at this moment discovers unexpectedly that the situation must be given thought.'

> *Stage 2.* All the time, in 'the period of hesitation' (as I call it), the baby holds his body still (but not rigid). Gradually he becomes brave enough to let his feelings develop, and then the picture changes quite quickly. The moment at which this first phase changes into the second is evident, for the child's acceptance of the reality of desire for the spatula is heralded by a change in the inside of the mouth, which becomes flabby, while the tongue looks thick and soft, and saliva flows copiously. . . .
>
> I have frequently made the experiment of trying to get the spatula to the infant's mouth during the stage of hesitation I find that it is impossible during this stage to get the spatula to the child's mouth apart from the exercise of brutal strength. . . .
>
> The baby now seems to feel that the spatula is in his possession, perhaps in his power, certainly available for the purposes of self-expression. He bangs with it on the table or on a metal bowl which is nearby on the table, making as much noise as he can; or else he holds it to my mouth and to his mother's mouth, very pleased if we *pretend* to be fed by it. He definitely wishes us to *play* at being fed, and is upset if we should be so stupid as to take the thing into our mouths and spoil the game as a game.
>
> At this point, I might mention that I have never seen any evidence of a baby being disappointed that the spatula is, in fact, neither food nor a container of food.
>
> (Winnicott, 1941: 53–4)

If we make an analogy from this to a baby's use of the spoon, we can see how necessary are the stages through which the baby comes to feel that the spoon is his for the taking. The spoon that is an extension of mother becomes a spoon that is a symbol of the baby's own agency.

Conclusion

In this paper, we have seen some of the difficulties in setting up a feeding relationship and the way in which emotional distance is represented in physical terms. Working in the baby clinic of a GP practice, I have heard from doctors and health visitors of how most infants with feeding problems have parents with eating disorders or other relationship problems. Research studies such as Stein's show that mothers with eating disorders often have problems in feeding their babies, and indeed public service advice to mothers makes this assumption in nationally distributed leaflets. A key element in a difficult feeding relationship may be the mother's intrusiveness.

Looking anecdotally at babies with early feeding problems, it would seem that some of the severe problems do carry on into the eating of solid foods. Other mothers may feel rescued by weaning from an unmanageable intimacy in early feeding. Now being explored is the continuity of infant feeding problems into adult eating disorders. Skuse suggests that the preoccupation with body shape of the young adult is a very separate causation.

Stein et al., looking from the adult with eating problems to the effect on her baby, ask what the relationship between the maternal eating disorder, maternal depression, and the baby's feeding disturbance consists of. Do the parental symptoms impinge directly on the child, or more subtly through the parent-infant interaction? They conclude that '[i]t would thus appear that a general difficulty with feeding is a more important mechanism in the transmission of disturbance rather than a direct effect of the mother's psychopathology' (1996).

Where does this lead us to direct our clinical energies? A recent Parent-Infant Workshop on 'Feeding Problems' at the Tavistock brought up an argument about whether psychotherapeutic work needed to take place around observation of actual feeds and mealtimes, or whether our usual relationship work is sufficient. Pinheiro (1993) states: 'Families under going the stress of struggling with a feeding problem, seem to be more effectively helped in the long run when these difficulties are seen in the context of their relationships.' Perhaps the key here is psychosis: where anxiety is replaced by inappropriate, even bizarre acts, in a feeding situation, then concrete work in the home may be indicated. Videos can also bridge these two kinds of intervention. Whatever route we choose, it is essential to remember that the major cause of the kind of feeding that results in a withholding of food from the infant is undoubtedly the experience by the parent of neglect, deprivation, and hunger in all its meanings, in their own childhood.

References

Bick, E. (1964). 'Notes on infant observation in psychoanalytic training'. *International Journal of Psycho-Analysis*, 45: 558–66.

Boddy, J. M., & Skuse, D. (1994). 'Annotation: The process of parenting in failure to thrive'. *Journal of Child Psychology and Psychiatry*, 35 (3): 401–24.

Bollas, C. (1987). *The Shadow of the Object: Psychoanalysis of the Unthought Known*. London: Free Association Books.

Briggs, S. (1997). *Growth and Risk in Infancy*. London: Jessica Kingsley.

Daws, D. (1993). 'Feeding problems and relationship difficulties: Therapeutic work with parents and infants'. *Journal of Child Psychotherapy*, 19 (2): 69–83.

Evans-Morris, S. (1977). 'Interpersonal aspects of feeding problems'. In: J. M. Wilson (Ed.), *Oral Motor Function and Dysfunction in Children*. Chapel Hill: University of North Carolina, pp. 106–22.

Fraiberg, S., Adelson, E., & Shapiro, V. (1980). 'Ghosts in the nursery: A psychoanalytic approach'. In: S. Fraiberg (Ed.), *Clinical Studies in Infant Mental Health*. London: Tavistock.

Guedeney, A. (1995). 'Kwashiorkor, depression and attachment disorders'. Letter in *The Lancet*, 346 (11 November): 1293.

Health Education Authority. (1995/6). *New Birth to Five*. London: HEA.

Hopkins, J. (1994). 'Therapeutic interventions in infancy: Two contrasting cases of persistent crying'. *Psychoanalytic Psychotherapy*, 8: 141–52.

Hopkins, J. (1996). 'The dangers and deprivations of too-good mothering'. *Journal of Child Psychotherapy*, 22 (3): 407–22.

Miller, R. L., Rustin, M., Rustin, M., & Shuttleworth, J. (1989). *Closely Observed Infants*. London: Duckworth.

Moore, T., & Ucko, L. E. (1957). 'Night waking in early infancy'. *Archives of Disease in Early Childhood*, 32: 333–42.

Parker, N. (1993). 'How far is near enough: A waiting game'. *Journal of Child Psychotherapy*, 19 (2): 37–51.

Pinheiro, M. (1993). 'A clinical study of early feeding difficulties: Risk and resilience in early mismatches within parent-infant relationships'. *Psychoanalytic Observational Studies*. Tavistock Clinic/University of East London.

Pollitt, E., Gilmore, M., & Valcarcel, M. (1978). 'Early mother-infant interaction and somatic growth'. *Early Human Development*, I: 325–36.

Ravenscroft, K., & Williams, G. (Eds.). (1997). *Feeding Difficulties in Childhood and Eating Disorders in Adolescence*. New York: Jason Aronson.

Selwyn, R. (1993). 'Psychodynamic aspects of failure to thrive: A case study'. *Journal of Child Psychotherapy*, 19 (2): 85–100.

Shapiro, V., Fraiberg, S., & Adelson, E. (1980). 'Billy: Infant-parent psychotherapy on behalf of a child in a critical nutritional state'. In: S. Fraiberg (Ed.), *Clinical Studies in Infant Mental Health*. London: Tavistock.

Skuse, D. (1993). 'Identification and management of problem eaters'. *Archives of Disease in Childhood*, 69: 604–8.

Skuse, D., & Wolke, D. (1992a). 'The nature and consequences of feeding problems in infancy'. In: P. Cooper & A. Stein (Eds.), *Feeding Problems and Eating Disorders in Children and Adolescents, Monographs in Clinical Paediatrics No 5*. Philadelphia: Harwood Academic Publishers.

Skuse, D., & Wolke, D. (1992b). 'The management of infant feeding'. In: P. Cooper & A. Stein (Eds.), *Feeding Problems and Eating Disorders in Children and Adolescents, Monographs in Clinical Paediatrics No 5*. Philadelphia: Harwood Academic Publishers.

Stein, A., Murray, L., Cooper, P., & Fairburn, C. G. (1996). 'Infant growth in the context of maternal eating disorders and maternal depression: A comparative study'. *Psychological Medicine*, 26: 569–74.

Stein, A., Woolley, H., Cooper, S. D., & Fairburn, C. G. (1994). 'An observational study of mothers with eating disorders and their infants'. *Journal of Child Psychology/Psychiatry*, 35: 733–48.

Stern, D. (1985). *The Interpersonal World of the Infant*. New York: Basic Books.

Trevarthan, C., & Hubley, P. (1978). 'Secondary intersubjectivity: Confidence, confiding and acts of meaning in the first year'. In: A. Lock (Ed.), *Action, Gesture, Symbol. The Emergence of Language*. New York: Academic Press.

Winnicott, D. W. (1941). 'The observation of infants in a set situation'. In: *Collected Papers: Through Paediatrics to Psychoanalysis*. London: Tavistock, 1958.

Winnicott, D. W. (1968). 'Breast-feeding as communication'. In: C. Winnicott, R. Shepherd, & M. Davis (Eds.), *Babies and Their Mothers*. London: Free Association Books, 1987.

Winnicott, D. W. (1971). 'Transitional objects and transitional phenomena'. In: *Playing and Reality*. London: Tavistock.

Wolke, D. (1996). 'Failure to thrive: The myth of maternal deprivation syndrome'. *The Signal, Newsletter of WAIMH*, 4 (3 & 4).

Part 3

Child psychotherapy

The frame and the setting

8 Consent in child psychotherapy

The conflicts for child patients, parents, and professionals

Originally published in the Journal of Child Psychotherapy (1986, Vol. 12, No. 1) *and given previously as a paper at a Symposium on 'Ethics' at the British Psychological Society's Conference, Warwick, April 1984.*

Samantha, a nine-year-old patient, fell asleep during a session. I let her sleep for a few minutes, then woke her, and sat next to her as she collected herself. It was nearly time to go, and I talked briefly of what I felt was her depression and her need to block out the pain of what we had earlier talked about in the session.

Two hours later, Samantha's mother, Mrs. H., phoned and asked, 'Did you hypnotize Samantha?'. The unexpectedness of the question, about a technique so outside my own practice of psychotherapy, nearly prompted me into a facetious reply, but in fact I answered seriously that I had not done so, that I did not know how to hypnotise, that, as far as I knew, no-one in our building used hypnosis, and that if it were used on children it would be with parents' knowledge and consent. Mrs. H. had only my word to go on but appeared satisfied by this interchange. The question remains, how is a responsible parent to evaluate what goes on between a professional and their child, when the professional insists on working in privacy and confidentiality that excludes the parent?

In the H. family's case, the difficulty was real. Samantha was referred for depression, which had started at the time of her father's death. Mrs. H. quarrelled with the clinic psychiatrist working with herself and refused to go on seeing him. She had been unable to let him raise the question of the loss of her husband. However, she was so anxious for Samantha to continue therapy that we agreed to do so, with many misgivings about working without close contact with a parent. Our misgivings were soon justified. It was obvious that, without the chance to check with us personally at the clinic, Mrs. H. was doing her checking outside. Conversations with a psychologist uncle prompted Samantha to say to me, 'Harold Lloyd isn't approved of.' An imaginative leap I was

DOI: 10.4324/b23125-11

rather proud of prompted me to ask, 'Do you mean Sigmund Freud?' She did mean Freud and was conveying to me the doubts in her family circle about the theories and techniques I might be subjecting her to.

From my point of view, working so one-sidedly was painfully limiting. Mrs. H. and Samantha had never been able to talk together about their bereavement and it felt as though both hoped father would come back. I had Mrs. H.'s permission to talk about it with Samantha but Samantha could hardly bear me to do so in this vacuum. For several of her once weekly visits, she engaged me in a game of hide and seek. The lost person she was trying to find was perhaps her father and also her mother of happier times. I was then struck by the 'babyish' quality of the game. She was playing, not as a nine-year-old but like a very small child. I said I thought she was trying to get back to be the little girl she was before her father's death. Samantha was shocked by this remark. She went white, sat down at the other side of the room, and remained silent for the rest of the session. I was worried about this reaction and thought she might not be able to come back to me. In fact, she came back the next time as though relieved of a burden. She became much more able to talk to me, and to listen to what I said and, in the session where she fell asleep, had talked openly of her grief at the loss of her father.

You can see that when Mrs. H. put her question, 'Did you hypnotize Samantha?' she was in an unusually vulnerable position, isolated from the clinic, without an experience of therapy for herself that would have given her a cross-bearing on what might be happening between Samantha and me. But we should not dismiss this question as coming from an awkward parent. The usefulness of all extreme reactions is in making us look at the universal elements they expose. I think that all parents, however cooperative, grateful or well-informed, have some version of the question, 'Did you hypnotize her?' to put to us. Perhaps the crucial function of any such question is to remind the professional, 'I am the parent, and I have a right to ask questions and be answered.'

Professionals have a need of such reminders. Listen to this unblushing account by Charlotte Bronte. In 'Jane Eyre,' the governess says of her pupil Adéle,

> My pupil was a lively child, who had been spoilt and was sometimes wayward; but as she was committed entirely to my care, and no injudicious interference from any quarter ever thwarted my plans for her improvement; she soon forgot her little freaks and became obedient and teachable.

We design our professional trainings to help curb such omnipotent feelings within ourselves. An intolerance of being thwarted is an excessive way of describing it, but perhaps we all have moments in professional life of still wishing we could do it all our own way. James Anthony, in his paper 'Other People's Children,' (1958) warns us of the dangers. He tells us always to remember that we are dealing with other people's children. Let me give you a list of some of the points he has italicised in this paper.

1. *They have been brought up in quite the wrong way.*
2. *Our own way is always the right way.*
3. *Other people's children are difficult.*
4. *We always want to alter other people's children.*
5. *There is a mother inside every child with whom we have to cope.*
6. *There are no deep taboos or incest barriers to protect other people's children from our sexuality.*
7. *We often tend to use other people's children to act out our problems.*

How do we use these thoughts? We have all thought of the complex issues involved in informing parents sufficiently so that they can validly give consent to their child's therapy. We have thought of the subtle questions of how capable the child is of giving his own consent. We agonise over how to proceed when the parents' consent or lack of it is at variance with the child's own position. What Anthony makes us look at is the professional's battle with the child's internalised parent. How does a parent give consent to that?

Usually when a child is referred for therapy and parents give consent, the therapy is thought of as an extension of the parents' own good care for that child; the therapist is providing a particular professional skill at the request of the parents, on behalf of their child. Sometimes, however, therapy is part of a combined rescue operation by a network of professionals. It is believed that not enough good parenting has been given to the child, and psychotherapy is relied on to provide one aspect of what is missing.

The paradox that Anthony points out to us is that the more that good parenting is lacking, the more the child in substitute care will resist the imposition of a substitute parent for his own imperfect one. Anthony says:

> To my way of thinking, surrogation is a measure of failure in casework. The more complete it is, in taking over the child, excluding contact with the parents, altering the child to our own image and likeness, bringing it up differently – the more is the child psychologically orphaned.

Anthony is warning us of the dangers of an extreme position. More usually we see ourselves in partnership with the parents of children we are concerned with.

Let us go back to the conversation between Mrs. H. and myself. It seemed that her question contained several layers of anxiety. What it really meant included, 'Are you qualified for what you do?' and, 'Are you taking advantage of my child's vulnerability?' I did not consciously work this out while replying to her, but my words seem to have answered her anxiety at this level.

A principle emerges from this. Patients or their parents give consent to treatment of all kinds in return for a promise from us that we have an ethical code that can be spelt out and that we keep to. More important is that his giving of consent is only the minimal basis on which a therapeutic intervention can begin to be set up. Real useful consent is part of an ongoing relationship between patient, or patient and family, and the therapist. Looking up 'consent' in the Oxford Dictionary, one finds a variety of meanings ranging from acquiescence and compliance towards what is suggested by another, to 'agreement in feeling, sympathy, accord.' It seems to me that consent in therapy must move along the range of these concepts to be of any use.

Consent is therefore not a once-for-all interchange of a formal and legal nature; it is an ongoing agreement of mutual interest. The wish for the therapy to take place does not come one-sidedly from a therapist and be agreed to by the consumer. If the active wish to make use of therapy is not also in the patient, at some level, then therapeutic change is unlikely to occur.

I began with a child patient's parent and her need to keep on checking what was going on in her child's therapy. Let us now look at it from the position of a child. How does a child start to give consent to his own treatment?

A four-year-old boy lined up with his mother and brother for all three to be vaccinated before going overseas. He said to the (somewhat annoyed) doctor, 'If it hurts I'll tell the police.' Although his mother had given her consent for him to be vaccinated, he was stating the inviolability of his own small body and backing it up by reference to a supreme authority. He was stating the limits of his consent.

An eight-year-old psychotherapy patient, Wayne, came into a session saying to me, 'You know you say I'm angry with you; well, I ain't.' I started to say something about him perhaps not actually being angry with me but he was bringing me angry feelings from somewhere else for us to think about. Wayne witheringly said, 'You're starting again.' Wayne was telling me, much more clearly than anything I was saying to him, that my comments were intrusive, incorrect, or in some other way unacceptable. He was not consenting to the way I was conducting the therapy.

Two children, both small and vulnerable, were each proclaiming their sense of self and their resistance to outside interference.

The way in which a child starts to build up a giving of consent to his therapy may turn out to be one of the main themes of the therapy. Giles, aged seven, and his mother were referred to the clinic in a mutual state of desperation. Both were depressed and very angry. I began to see Giles once weekly and his mother began therapy twice weekly with a very experienced colleague. At first, he sat in sullen silence, staring down at the table and kicking his legs against his chair. I did my best to interpret the anger and hopelessness of getting any help from me that I thought he was communicating. Then his mother told me that Giles hated the actual timing of his sessions – he arrived at school in the middle of assembly and was embarrassed by this. Therapy times are inconvenient for many children. Our working day coincides largely with the school day and out of school times are reserved for older children with exams in sight, or to fit in with working parents. Usually with younger children one hopes to work through the objections and find a time that feels least awkward to them. With Giles, I was unusually moved to offer an earlier, before school, time. The change in him was remarkable. He came willingly, brought small objects in his pockets, and put these on the table to show to me. He talked about these possessions and gradually also used the toys that I had provided for him. He began to talk about himself and his difficult family life.

Giles's father had left his mother when she was pregnant and gone to live abroad. His mother had brought him up valiantly on her own; she was successful in her own profession, but her long working hours were a strain on Giles and on herself. He resented an unrelenting timetable that meant he was looked after by others for some hours after school. In the first years of managing on her own, Giles's mother had little money to spend on child-minding, and her own stress made it difficult for her to find consistent arrangements that really worked. Giles felt he was being dumped with no reference to his own needs or wishes.

I realised then that his therapy had been experienced by Giles as the same sort of arrangement – made by adults for their own convenience, with no reference to him. I hope that eventually I would have guessed at this, even without changing his time, and been able to use it as a communication of his experience of life. As it was, my change of time allowed him to start using the therapy in an easy, direct way. What allowed this radical change was not that I had proved better than his mother in offering a time that suited him, but that his mother had managed to communicate to me that there were aspects of timing that were intolerable to Giles. Within the safety of this partnership, Giles was able to tell me of his feeling of worthlessness at being pushed around. His fury with his mother abated and as he became more cooperative, his mother could look after him better. The therapy perhaps offered some aspects of a parental partnership to Giles's mother: Her therapist and I became in different degrees Giles's missing father and gave her some of the protection and support she needed to feel her own value as a good mother.

Giles's consent to therapy represented his consent to his mother bringing him up in the best way available to her, and we were able to use the concept of this some years later.

Giles and his mother came back to me recently to discuss whether Giles should go to boarding school at the approaching age of 13. There was an understanding in the extended family that he should do so and relatives had offered to pay for the school. Giles's mother was anxious to work out whether this felt like an opportunity to Giles, or a rejection of him from herself. I suggested that they go home, and in privacy talk through together the experience of Giles's early years – of how their mutual difficulties had arisen and how they had reached some understanding about them. I felt that if they could clear this first, there would be no 'hidden agenda' of past mutual reproach in making their new decision. Giles's mother managed with her now-adolescent son to tell him of the feelings she had had to face bringing him up on her own, of how her fury with her deserting husband had sometimes transferred onto him, and how her own professional ambitions had sometimes conflicted with her wish to devote herself to looking after him. With all this out in the open, they decided Giles should go to boarding school and I felt that Giles's consent to this was based on a genuine emotional freedom of choice.

Another case shows how lack of consent from a child and his father negated therapy. Hector was brought to me at seven for bedwetting. This again was a child being brought up by his mother, although father, who had remarried, lived near and was in close touch with his son. It emerged that mother was eager for therapy for Hector and for herself. Father visited the clinic at our request but presented a bland and patronising attitude to my colleague and me. My colleague helped mother with her over-involvement with her son, and with the nappies he was still bizarrely wearing. Hector seemed blandly unaware that there was a problem. First, I interpreted the internal conflicts that I thought might be the personal reasons for this particular child's lack of control. Then my colleague, an experienced behaviour therapist, attempted to set out a structure in which Hector could achieve continence. She and I met together with Hector and his mother to work out some of the family dynamics involved. I experienced a range of feelings about Hector's bedwetting – sympathy for his predicament, excitement at the thought of helping him change, exasperation at his lack of change, a desire to control him, to force him to change, fury when he did not comply, and a feeling of being 'shown up' by my therapeutic failure. Hector seemed little affected by any of these feelings. I was having them on my own. It occurred to my colleague and me that it mattered little whether we tried psychotherapy, behaviour therapy, or family therapy. We had of course urged the 'bell and pad' method on Hector and his mother at each stage of our intervention, and the failure of this well-tried cure of the symptom itself should have alerted us. We realised that Hector was bringing an important part of himself to the clinic, his identification with a father who was unwilling to look at problems. Interpretation of this was not likely to be welcomed.

It is crucial in Hector's case to distinguish between lack of consent to therapy and resistance within therapy. In all of us, whether in therapy or not, there is a degree of resistance to change, a feeling that the pain involved in making change is far worse than the pain involved in keeping even inadequate functioning going. Resistance in therapy is a way of taking account of this pain, and patients who have an overall wish to function in a more healthy way use their resistance as part of their struggle towards change. In Hector's case, there appeared to be no such struggle.

To go back to the dictionary, consent in physiological terms means 'sympathy between one organ or part of the body and another.' In a dynamic process of psychotherapy, consent is hard-won as unconscious and conscious parts of the mind struggle with each other to achieve this sympathy.

I hope I am building up a picture of the intertwining of parents' and child's consent. Sometimes parents bring a child to the clinic and then are in conflict with each other about whether the child needs therapy. I often feel in these cases that they are holding two valid aspects of expectation of therapy, or indeed of how disturbed their child is. I suggest to them that each try to hold on to their own position, and put it together with the other's, so that, for example, an over-optimistic feeling that therapy will take over and cure all problems, put together with a belief that the child will 'just grow out of it,' might result in a combined moderate view that therapy could facilitate normal development.

Sometimes conflict about therapy simply illustrates acute marital conflict, which includes conflict about what is in the children's interests. The child is then in a dilemma: if he is offered therapy he can only please one parent. One patient poignantly solved this problem. Diane was in a family where the parents were in a state of continual bitter warfare. They rarely spoke to each other and automatically attacked when they did so. Their son was at a board-ing school for maladjusted children and mother saw the clinic social worker weekly. Diane had somehow been slipped into therapy without father's proper consent. Diane used her therapy as a lifeline to look at her position, caught between her parents, able seldom to please either. Father protested at her ther-apy continuing, and we had a meeting of the social worker and mother, a male psychiatrist to give father some masculine support, Diane, and myself. Faced with the conflicting suggestions from father that she should stop therapy, and from mother that she should continue as infinitely as mother longed for her own therapy to continue, Diane herself came up with the proposal that she should come fortnightly. This was agreed to with relief all round.

Diane had previously used her therapy with me in a tentative way, and there had been many silences while she did obsessional repetitive drawings. She now used every moment to the full, confiding in me much more openly the ten-sions of her family life. I said that I thought her parents' conflict about therapy had in fact connected with conflicting feelings in herself about it. Now that she came fortnightly, perhaps the week she did not come contained the negative feelings; the one where she did come she could proceed with the positive ones. If I had missed this split and felt myself only to be the helpful therapist sup-porting a vulnerable child with her feelings about difficult parents outside the therapy room, I would also have missed the chance for her to look directly at these negative feelings and experience them in regard to myself.

Particularly when a child's real life contains much conflict, it is essential for the therapist to remain clear that his job is to help the child contain conflicting feelings without the therapist being impelled to rush into action. Where parents are in conflict about therapy, it is of vital importance not to assume that the par-ent in favour of therapy is the one with the true interests of the child at heart.

There are times also when I stipulate that my consent to therapy is needed. Leo, an 11-year-old boy, came to me in a panic about going to school. His father had died suddenly a couple of years earlier and the shock of his death was still acute. Leo had started to feel ill at about the second anniversary of the death and the trouble about going to school dated from then. Leo's misery was genuine but he also seemed to be exploiting his mother and the rest of the family into seeing him as interesting and special. I felt that if I started to see Leo straight away, with the intention of relieving his immediate emotional distress and then easing him back into school, we could find it taking months to get him back. I therefore offered to see him twice weekly, on condition that he returned to school first. Leo was horrified at my obtuseness and hardness, but his mother, supported by the social worker, and I stood firm. Leo then quickly got the point that, having made his concession by going back to school, he was free to use therapy for as long as it was dynamically useful to him in working out his problems, including his conflicting feelings about the father who had died. School phobic patients may worry that getting over their symptoms means the end of their therapy. Leo was able to avoid this dilemma and continued therapy weekly for over a year. He became a happier and physically more robust-looking boy.

I have described how consent of parents and children is an ongoing process. If the therapist is in some sort of contact with parents, how is the confidentiality of the therapy preserved? Further to this, a child in therapy not only has parents, he has a network of schools and, if there have been difficulties over a period, perhaps other agencies. The therapist who knows the child so well is tempted to be part of this network and to use her knowledge for the child's benefit. Furthermore, if she is not an available and visible part of this network, hostility may well build up from the other agencies. They may wonder, as did Samantha's mother, what this non-visible person is up to with their child. The dangers are, then, if the therapist is an active part of a network, all doing things for the child, will she lose her ability to sit down and painstakingly go through feelings with the child that are too painful, too precarious to be expressed other than in private?

Douglas was a charming, verbal eight-year-old who was excluded from his primary school for disturbed behaviour. He had therapy with me at our Day Unit and was able to verbalise his problems. His insight was so much greater than his ability to control his behaviour that I was stung into saying to him, 'If you understand your feelings so well, why can't you behave better?' When he was ten, he was taken rather gingerly back into a normal primary school. He wished at that point to stop coming to therapy, but the school refused to take him unless he continued. Having been very eager to use therapy, he now became very sour about being labelled by me and the school as still being a 'problem child.' I countered by talking about his unrealistic wish to leave all his problems instantly behind in me. The school were perhaps over observant of Douglas; he felt they were always picking on him. I offered, with Douglas's permission, to visit his school and discuss the situation with the teachers. I felt that this was helpful in getting the teachers to anticipate that Douglas might need a longer period of time to feel properly settled in the school and that his brief outbursts of violent behaviour were not their failure. Meanwhile, I discussed all these outbursts with Douglas as from the school's point of view, pointing out that they only had the evidence of his actual behaviour to go on in forming their present opinion of him. I had obviously been taking my role of referee too far and was neglecting to keep in touch with Douglas's own feelings about himself. He said to me, 'I come to therapy to say what I think, not for you to make up your own mind.' This paper has aimed to show how the giving of consent to therapy in effect becomes the building up of a consensus, or sympathy between therapist and patient. The paradox that emerges is that this consent is based on patients and therapists working upon their personal conflicts and resistances. In fact, in this paper we started with the socio-legal concept of consent but have traced its functioning in several individual cases. From this point of view, we see that consent, or lack of it, is one facet of individual resistance. This may be a valuable or deleterious process. Whichever of these, it is a vital aspect of the dynamic conflicts which can assail anyone's life.

One final point. Consent to therapy is not consent for action. In this, the difficulty for the therapist is in remaining able to hold on to what the patient has consented to, that is, to work on the pain of his conflicts within the boundaries of this consensus. Taking action on behalf of the patient may often seem to be a useful common sense procedure. Or it may be an acting out by the therapist of the conflict expressed by the patient. Doing and acting out one aspect of a conflicting situation effectively stops the therapist from feeling on behalf of the patient what pain an impulsive action is trying to evade. The action then negates the patient's chance to bear his pain himself and make his own resolution. Douglas reminded me that I had overstepped what he had consented to in our work together and that I was evading the work of exploration of pain by my interventions.

By recognising these dilemmas within ourselves, we are strengthened when dealing with such issues in others. Where parents may be in conflict against a school, against a diagnosis, against a recommendation, action is usually necessary. What is also vital is giving these parents the opportunity to look first at their distress at their child's difficulties or handicaps before expecting any consent to what we have to offer. Understanding how action can be a flight from distress allows us to speculate whether agencies that urge parents to fight for their children's rights are doing them a real service, or perhaps robbing them of a chance to first bear, and thus manage, the pain of their child's limitations, before finding the best provision for their child's particular needs.

Shakespeare knew the need for grief to be fully experienced before action can be appropriately taken, and the fallacy of believing that precipitate action can cut short mourning. I end with a quotation from 'Macbeth' (IV, iii). This deals with the bereavement of actual death but illuminates the issue of dealing with any loss. Macduff is told that his wife and children have been slain; Malcolm urges him.

"Be comforted.
Let's make us medicines of our great revenge to cure this deadly grief,"
and further provokes him with,
"Dispute it like a man."
Macduff replies,
"I shall do so,
But I must also feel it as a man."

References

Anthony, J. (1958). Other People's Children in *Children in Care*. Ed. R. J. N. Tod. London: Longman.

Bronte, C. Jane Eyre, Chapter XII. (1984). Penguin English Library, London.

Shakespeare, W. Macbeth (1623). *Shakespeare's Complete Works* (1984). Oxford: Oxford University Press.

9 Resistance and co-operation

The need for both. A further study of psychotherapy in a Day Unit

Originally published in the Journal of Child Psychotherapy (1983, Vol. 9, No. 2) *and given previously as a paper at the Surrey C.G.C's Inter-Clinic Conference, July 1983.*

I work in a psychiatric Day Unit attached to a Child Guidance Clinic, officially a hospital school. I have described elsewhere (1977) the particular issues involved in working in individual psychotherapy with children in the place where the child spends his schooldays. In this paper, my interest is in looking at how psychotherapy fits into the institution. I give a clinical example of a case where I felt I could attempt psychotherapy with a disturbed little girl with the backing and support of the Day Unit. Although I give much specific detail of how the professions relate in one particular institution, I hope that anyone involved in the setting up of therapy for children will be reminded of their own relevant network, be it families, GPs, teachers at ordinary schools.

The Day Unit differs essentially from, for example, a school for maladjusted children, in that it is an NHS facility with a consultant psychiatrist as head of the Unit. There is a part-time psychiatric staff of four, the psychiatrist, a social worker, educational psychologist, and child psychotherapist. However, the Unit is run as a school by a teacher-in-charge who is one of three full-time Inner London Education Authority (ILEA) teachers with one part-time ILEA remedial teacher, and three full-time nursery assistants employed by the NHS. The other staff are a full-time secretary/administrator, a caretaker, and a cook, all NHS employees.

The Unit was founded some 15 years ago by staff of the parent clinic, and seen then, among its other uses, as a Unit where children in therapy could be placed. Over the years, it has been seen by referrers in the community, psychiatrists in other Child Guidance Clinics, teachers, educational psychologists, E.W.O.s, etc., as a place to refer children who for many disparate reasons have broken down in their normal schools. These are children who may or may not benefit from psychotherapy. The Unit offers a relatively short-term placement averaging two years, and during these years it is hoped that the child will

DOI: 10.4324/b23125-12

be able to recover from the personal breakdown or disintegration that often accompanies the breakdown of their school placement. That is, with clinic referrals, a child and his family may have to concentrate on and exaggerate their difficulties in order to precipitate the help that is needed.

When a child is placed in the Day Unit, there is often an enormous feeling of relief that the difficulties of managing in a large school are no longer there. Although of course this may be something of a 'honeymoon' experience, the relief of not having to deal with a large complicated institution remains, and children can begin to sort out their problems in a small supportive unit.

The average two-year stay allows time for a child to recover from this first stage of breakdown, and for a therapeutic reintegrative process to happen before the child is referred on to a long-term placement, either back into the normal school system or into special education of some kind, day or residential, or into residential hospital placement. The range of problems dealt with at the Day Unit is very wide, and providing a suitable therapeutic experience for all these children adds to the variety and interest of working there. It adds also to the tensions and conflicts for staff in trying to decide what is best for children with such different needs.

The Day Unit is divided into three small groups, roughly according to age, each taken by a teacher and assistant. The idea of having two members of staff to each group is intrinsic to the Unit. Each pair provides a model of a parental couple, irrespective of their particular sex, a model of a couple working together, using individual differences and characteristics in partnership for the benefit of the child. As well as acting as a model the couple are a support for each other; when absorbing the projections of a very disturbed child, it is essential to be able to catch the eye of a partner who is not being overwhelmed by these projections. The teacher who is with the child can then perhaps manage to stay emotionally with him and contain the projections without being tempted to fling them back at the child.

This brings us to a definition of what constitutes 'therapy' in a therapeutic setting. The Day Unit is thought of as a therapeutic Unit. The three groups are run as classroom groups and the children have school lessons and other school-based activities and outings for much of the day. Some, but not all, of the children have individual remedial teaching, and some have individual psychotherapy. How is it decided who will have this, and how does it fit in with the work of the Unit as a whole? Like the partnership of teacher and assistant in each group, is there a partnership between the group's teacher couple and the individual therapist that some children have?

The ambience of the Day Unit is psychoanalytically informed; at its simplest this means that all the staff have a knowledge that the unconscious exists, that disturbed children are in the grip of unresolved unconscious conflicts, and that the way to help them lies in providing a contained understanding structure where they can express these conflicts and work through them.

This working through can be at two levels, one where the conflict remains unconscious but is responded to appropriately and, secondly, where connections are made for the child so that the unconscious becomes to differing degrees conscious. Our everyday problem is, how much of each of these processes is relevant for any particular child, which is more therapeutically effective and who should do it? Is interpretation the province only of the psychotherapist or should the teacher on the spot say the obvious and give the sort of psychic first-aid that some children seem to call out for? If teacher does make an interpretation, can the child actually bear it in the classroom without privacy, or alternatively will it feel as though permission has been given to use the classroom as an individual psychotherapy setting? Let us go back to the reasons for referral to the Day Unit; these seem to come at two different levels of conceptualising a problem. One kind of referral comes from Child Guidance Clinics where a psychiatric assessment has already been made that the child is in need of individual psychotherapy, and may already be in therapy at that clinic; the other broad category is simply that the child is no longer able to maintain daily attendance at a local normal or special school and is felt to be in need of the special attention that a small Unit can offer.

In all these cases, a rigorous diagnostic procedure is offered to each child by the Day Unit. The child and family are seen by the psychiatrist, educational psychologist, and social worker and by the teacher-in-charge and the teacher in the group the child might be taken into. This diagnostic procedure serves to assess the suitability or otherwise of the child for the Day Unit, and vice versa. It can also serve as a consultation by an experienced team in formulating the nature of an elusive problem and suggesting other more suitable facilities. Offering of a place to a child depends on the feeling that he will personally make use of the Unit, and also on the balance of the appropriate age groups at any one moment. It seems to work best to have a variety of personalities and problems in each group, so that any one does not consist entirely of, say, withdrawn non-speaking children, or conversely of acting-out impulsive ones.

This diagnostic and selection procedure determines who is felt to be suitable for the Day Unit, that is who could make good use of its therapeutic environment as a whole. How then does psychotherapy fit in?

Paradoxically for a therapeutic unit committed to work psychodynamically, it does not always augur well for psychotherapy already to have been recommended at the time of referral to the Unit. When a child is already in psychotherapy or when there is a strong expectation that psychotherapy will set up when the child starts at the Unit, a feeling of resistance to the therapy may build up in the Day Unit. Where does this feeling stem from and what does it mean? It is easy to dismiss such feelings as resistance to psychoanalytic thinking, to a difficulty in sharing a child with the therapist, to envy of the specific skill of the therapist, or of the confidential intimate relationship between child and therapist. Of course, some elements of all this may exist, in fact perhaps they should exist. If psychotherapy is the rigorous, disturbing, absorbing experience we claim it to be for therapist and patient alike, can we expect the colleagues close at hand to this process to confine themselves to an absent-mindedly benevolent support? Strong feelings will be aroused, not all of them friendly, and this is part of our shared working situation.

I think we should take this as seriously as Freud found he had to take the resistance to psychoanalysis of his patients. We should take it that resistance is not an awkward phenomenon that can be ignored, reasoned away, or removed by high-powered trickery. Resistance in a patient is a resistance to change in the personality. It shows us that the pain involved in making a change is felt at the time to be even greater than the pain involved in keeping inadequate functioning going. The psychoanalyst or therapist who can help a patient successfully negotiate this change is the one who can remain with it and see the struggle itself as the instrument of change. The resistance that some members of a multi-professional working unit sometimes show towards psychotherapy must be equally taken seriously as an intrinsic aspect of the dynamic working of the Unit, and we must learn from it.

It must not become polarised so that some individuals feel themselves pushed into the position of being anti-therapy and others to have an unrealistically optimistic expectation of it. It is more helpful to acknowledge the ambivalence about therapy that is within us all, even therapists (or even especially therapists). Therapeutic zeal is more credible when tempered with a little depressive doubt. Alternatively, we cannot allow this resistance to block the setting up of psychotherapy – to act as a veto. It is only valuable as a dimension of the struggle towards change.

Psychotherapy in a therapeutic environment represents an essence, a distillation of the work going on every day within this environment. The sessions of individual psychotherapy may be an enhanced experience inside the therapy room of what goes on outside it – the child brings the same sort of play material to the therapy, makes the same sort of confidences about himself to the therapist as he does to his teacher. The difference is that with the teacher he gets a broad acceptance and understanding of himself and his conflicts; with the therapist he may get a specific and detailed verbal interpretation which helps him make a link between his conscious and unconscious knowledge of himself. Both teacher and therapist may be efficiently helping him move on to another level of self-knowledge and ability to use his intellectual and emotional facilities more effectively.

In other children, the use of classroom and therapy is apparently more separate. The child may focus bringing his unconscious conflicts into the therapy sessions and be free to use the classroom more straightforwardly and concentrate on learning. One patient of mine, a little boy of six, was observed by his teachers to shake himself each time he came back into the classroom after his therapy session. He seemed to need to shake off the internal preoccupations of his therapy in order to re-enter the everyday external world.

A child like this shows how painful the transition can be from inner to outer reality. We all know the children who cannot let themselves make this difficult transition and keep the boundaries intact; they noisily come to and from their therapy, they disturb the classroom before and particularly after, their sessions.

By not knowing when to start and when to stop their session, they never fully experience being alone with the therapist in the seclusion of the therapy room. They break the confidentiality of their own therapy as though the drama around it mattered more to them than the therapy itself. The pain for this sort of child in moving in and out of his therapy is often projected into the adults around and becomes dramatised by them. When teachers and therapist feel themselves to be in conflict with each other about therapy it is worth examining it in terms of conflicting feelings the child cannot hold inside himself.

Winnicott said something like, 'There is no such thing as a baby. Only a baby and its mother:' Perhaps also – there is no such thing as a child in therapy – only a child, its parents, and the therapist. In a Unit such as ours the support to a child in therapy may often be not the actual parents, but a parenting aspect of the teachers and other staff. A child cannot go off to therapy from a vacuum – even if he journeys himself he needs to be sent and received back by someone. If he is not, then the therapist may find himself inappropriately trying to fulfil aspects of a parental role, instead of being free to receive transference of feelings about parental figures. A patient of mine, an 11-year-old girl in care, was living in a children's home that was rapidly disintegrating and shortly afterwards closed. I was able to support a plan which enabled her to be eventually fostered. In the meantime, as I drove home after seeing her I had unfinished thoughts on the lines of 'Fostering is more use to children in care than psychotherapy.' My point is that it was not only this girl's parentlessness which gave rise to a sentimental fantasy from both her and myself that if only I would foster her all would be well. It was her lack of *substitute* parents, of someone to take immediate care of her and responsibility for her in a real way outside of the therapy that was so painfully obvious to us both.

In the Day Unit, it is often the teaching staff who provide support for the child in therapy. This can in some cases be the only support the child gets for his therapy. It sometimes seems worthwhile within the Unit to attempt therapy with children from disturbed families who would find it very difficult to support either emotionally or practically therapy at a clinic. It then becomes the Unit staff who offer the emotional containment and the assumption of an everyday knowledge of the child's state of emotional development. They do this instead of the parents. In other cases, the staff simply stand in for parents because they are present at the school and the parents are not. They send the child to his sessions and they receive him back, but it is as an extension of the parents' care for their child, not as a substitute for it.

If teaching staff in such a situation have a parental role to fill in the support of therapy, have they not also have some parental rights? This is an excessive way of stating it, perhaps, but I think it is unrealistic to expect enthusiastic support for therapy unless the staff members concerned have had some involvement in the process of deciding a child could benefit from therapy. It has been said that children have therapy because someone wants them changed. It may well be that children are referred because they are a nuisance to someone, even the referral of a quiet depressed child may be because it upsets someone to see him like that. What matters for us in this concept is that if someone wants a child changed then they know him as he is, the dissatisfaction with the child has a positive function and includes a relationship between referrer and child, something within the referrer connects with the child and feels all is not well. If this process has already happened and the child is already in therapy, staff may never feel so engaged with the therapy and may resent or question the need for it.

This process also holds in selection for the Unit. Teaching staff have told me how the method of admission to the Unit of one little boy, Mario, from a powerful but tragic family from abroad, had coloured their feeling about him in the classroom. This six-year-old boy, an obvious victim of circumstances, has a tiresomely imperious manner. His teachers have coped with much more difficult behaviour from the disturbed children they teach. It was they, not me, who made a link between their lack of sympathy with Mario's imperiousness and the high-handed way in which enthusiastic therapists and psychiatrists had eased his route from a teaching hospital to the Unit and five times a week analysis. Delicate negotiations had gone on with his capricious parents. Consultation within the Unit had been virtually nil. The normal admission procedure which allows two opportunities for the staff to consider a new entry had been curtailed and the teachers in the group never had the opportunity to make a place inside themselves for Mario.

We all know the disruption that premature births can cause to parents who had not quite got themselves ready; we know how the outcome of an adoption can be influenced by the way in which the introduction is handled and by how much preparation time the adoptive parents have had before they receive the baby. It is not far-fetched to suggest that professionals offering a child special care in a special unit need a recognised way of making room inside themselves for each new disturbed child who comes into the Unit. Leading on from this, I suggest that when a child enters therapy, a prerequisite is that the teachers who are intimately involved with him need to discover afresh for that child from within themselves the need for therapy.

The reality is not as piously cooperative as this might sound. A teacher may say, 'John is threatening the other children with the scissors. I think he needs therapy,' and the therapist reply, '*I* don't feel like seeing him if he is like that.' The serious issue behind this interchange is, 'Who is responsible for this child's aggression – can it be pushed on to the therapist or can classroom and therapy share the experience of it?' Similarly, can we share a child's depression? and, more seriously, the experience of a psychotic child? These last are the most tragic to deal with and the therapy of psychotic children remains a dilemma within our Unit. We have had several experiences where the pain of these children has become nakedly revealed. They have become apparently much more disturbed and the disturbance resounds through the Unit psychically as well as physically. Deeply felt and sincere differences of opinion among the professional staff about the validity of the position each time.

To redress the balance, in many of our cases psychotherapy is set up after we have all observed that a child is already benefiting from the general therapeutic setting of the Unit. In these cases, our expectation of what psychotherapy can achieve will be coloured by the therapeutic alliance the child has engaged in with the staff he already knows. The therapist thus builds on the goodwill other staff have created. One might expect goodwill to surround the therapy. Even so, through the most apparently tranquil therapy, we would do well not to forget the reverberances that run through each of us connected with the child. Therapy is going to stir up feelings, in the child, in the therapist, and in colleagues. A therapeutic unit is supposed to be able to stand such feelings. If we look at the setting for therapy with too much delicacy, we can find ourselves condoning our own laziness or moral cowardice.

In our Unit, I am the permanent psychotherapist and see two or three children at any one time. The psychiatrist also sees children and we have a trainee psychotherapist and a registrar who have training cases at the Unit. Some children may already be in therapy at an outside clinic, or our own clinic. Others are seen by therapists coming up to the Day Unit. We have increasingly found that in spite of the difficulties of organisation in having several therapists working in the Unit, this outweighs the disadvantages of having the therapy at a distance, even the short one to our own clinic. It seems as though the more a therapist can be a part of the Day Unit, the more they can have face-to-face contact with the staff working full-time in the Unit, the more the child's therapy is protected. Visiting therapists vary in style from those who can spare the time to have lunch or coffee at the Unit, or who *know* when the teacher has her break in order to phone her then; to those who apparently see themselves as autonomous and for example arrange holidays without enquiring how this relates to Day Unit breaks.

I hold occasional seminars, some with the therapists only, some with therapists and teachers together, where we hope to discuss the issues, to say to each other some of the things there is never time or occasion for in daily work. We often start with the specific technical problem of how a therapist takes a child from classroom to therapy room. The minutiae of detail of whether the therapist goes into the classroom, whether the teacher sends the child out over the threshold, and the many idiosyncratic variations that difficult children drive us to devise; these seem to me to sum up in a nutshell the basic problem – how does a child negotiate his way from teacher to therapist and how do we help him to do so? It is a wise therapist who does not attempt to start a child's session at a time when he is playing in the garden. If he is showing even a modicum of reluctance to come to his therapy the wide-open spaces literally put him beyond anyone's reach. He is too far away to feel the containment from either side, and no-one's job description includes running round the garden to fetch children for therapy. I mention this, obvious though it sounds, because I think the way we show mutual good faith is in the first place setting up practical arrangements that work. Times must be arranged that are mutually convenient, that acknowledge the importance of the school timetable and of the therapist's timetable, and of the experience for the child of when he comes out of the school routine and when he goes back into it.

This is our first provision. If we can do this within the very real limitations, then one enormous source of mutual irritation is gone. If the timing is badly wrong for the classroom then every time the therapist knocks and puts her head round the classroom door, the teacher will *not* feel that the therapy is an extension of her work with the child; she will feel it breaks into and diminishes the value of her work. A therapist fitting uncomfortably into the school timetable and rushing up the hill from another patient may not have the space and readiness to take in a child's disturbance. She will feel persecuted by both patient and institution.

If we get this very basic framework right and if therapists and teachers feel comfortable with each other, then both are in a better position to take on the child's projections. It often happens that once a child is in therapy, the severe states of being are much increased. The temptation is of course to attribute the pain of this to someone else. Therapists, teachers, parents, all feel that someone else is stirring up, or failing to contain aggression, depression, or whatever else is in question. Therapists are the most likely culprits and patients share this view. One articulate boy of nine assured me, 'You make my life a misery.' It is sometimes hard to hold on to the knowledge that it was someone's misery that *brought* them to therapy, and that competent therapy provides an opportunity to transfer onto the therapist the miseries and conflicts of his previous relationships and experience. This we find can take place most effectively *in* a separate, private, and confidential setting.

Here we have a dilemma. So far in this paper, I have described how I think that getting together to provide a protective network for a child's therapy is an important prerequisite. I have suggested that if therapist and teacher know each other face to face they are less likely to misinterpret the other's dealings with the child. The dilemma is this – if we take this too far and therapist and teacher understand each other too well – if they have too many dealings with each other, then there will be no space for the child's therapy. I repeat that therapy is essentially a private and confidential business, sometimes a lonely business. If all is shared then perhaps there will be nothing to share. Both therapist and teacher have to use their mutual goodwill to tolerate the point at which they can no longer work together. They have to tolerate for themselves a point of separation and they have to help the child cross the bridge from one to another and back again.

This does not mean each one abrogating his own area of authority. My colleague, Jo Jacobs, has pointed out to me that difficulty in defining boundaries can lead to diffidence on both sides. Neither wants to obtrude into the other's territory, and the child is left wondering to whom he belongs.

Because our colleagues in the classroom are themselves concerned to protect the confidentiality of the therapy, they may withdraw from action when the therapist appears. At one level I am talking about the occasional child who needs a firm physical handing over from teacher to therapist. More generally, there is implied a psychic handover, that is, an implicit understanding from teacher to child that she knows what sort of thing she is sending the child off to, and what sort of experience the child has had on coming back. Many of the children in our Unit cannot stand separations. The material of their therapy may be pervaded with them, and the comings and goings from therapy symbolise separation for them every time. If teacher and therapist can make an empathic leap with the child into the other's territory each way, then the child is helped to manage the dangers.

I said earlier that when we find ourselves in conflict about a child's therapy, the key is in the conflicting feelings within the child. It often appears that conflicts are expressed not by rows but by failures of communication. We are all guilty of these. What do they mean? The failures occur firstly in one professional failing to pass on some arrangement made in the course of their own work with the child, which affects other colleagues. More seriously, one part of the team finds itself making plans that affect the child's future without discussing these with other members of the team. We all do it. What possesses us? It seems to me that at these times we are overtaken by the projection of the child's anxieties, or someone else's anxiety about the child. If these anxieties only take account of one aspect of the child's needs, that is one aspect of conflicting feelings, then the worker may be swayed by the strength of this and act accordingly.

This sort of situation occurs at times in decisions about a child leaving the Unit. Often, it is impossible for us to have a consensus of opinion about the right time for a child to leave. The timescale for therapy is often much longer than the useful time a child can stay in the Unit. A feeling of movement in the child's life urges on a change of school; only the therapist wants more time to resolve infantile conflicts. One side feels the other is blinkered to the child's real interests. For many children, therapy is only possible within the framework of the Unit. When the natural momentum of the Unit's work comes to an end, or when with more disturbed children the Unit and often the home can no longer satisfactorily contain them, then it seems obvious on one level that the child should be placed elsewhere. It is ironical that the aspect of the Unit that is a holding for therapy can disappear at a moment when the therapist feels the child most needs a promise of continuity. Differing views of the child's needs seem irreconcilable, and the decisions we make seem arbitrary. Perhaps again we pick up the child's own panic about separation – difficulties in negotiating the way in which a child leaves the Unit may represent the enormous conflict within him and his readiness to leave. Between us, we hold the range of his feelings – even if he cannot, can we dare to put them together?

One child I had in therapy provides examples of many of the problems I have outlined. The problems of separation and the concept of privacy also prevailed. This is not a particularly successful case, but one of interest to me and members of staff, and contains many examples of how we have cooperated or not in the course of her therapy. The irreconcilable paradox is that by talking about this child I have broken the essence of the confidentiality that is one of my themes.

Josephine

I started to see Josephine once weekly after she had been one year in our Day Unit. She was an obviously disturbed, unhappy little girl of six, with a serious eye defect following a car-crash when she was aged two. Josephine was the fifth child in the family and had a brother a year younger than herself. This family was chaotic and there was much obvious stress. The older children had various artistic talents and were successful academically. Josephine had been excluded from her primary school for her unruly behaviour before coming to the Day Unit and her self-esteem was low. Josephine's therapy was set up by mutual agreement in the Unit. There was a feeling that she was responding well to the therapeutic environment of the Unit and was ready to take therapy 'on board.' I met her parents with the social worker *of* the Unit and found them in despair about their daughter. It seemed to me that they were so occupied with the problems of the family in general, and the severity of Josephine's disturbance, that the offer of therapy made little impact on them. In fact, I subsequently had very few dealings with her parents. They never initiated contact themselves, although they were always friendly when I spoke to them on the phone and agreed readily when I offered a second weekly session, a few weeks after we started.

I was a bit taken aback when I went up to them at a parents' evening, and they failed to recognise me. So with Josephine, it was very much her own teachers, and the Day Unit staff in general, with whom I discussed the progress of her treatment and her state of development. For example, when I offered a second session it was at the suggestion of her class teacher, who observed that a week was too long for her to wait between sessions.

In the first session her teacher, Mrs. D, offered, as she usually does, to accompany Josephine and me to my room. Josephine is the only child who has refused this offer – she made a pushing-away gesture with her hand and then walked to my room as though she knew the way. This was the first example for me of her constant determination to be in control. In the room, she dashed to a desk, opened a drawer, and was disconcerted to find it empty. I pointed out her own drawer of toys, opened ready for her in a chest of drawers at the other side of the room. She tried all the other drawers, found them to be locked, except for the top empty one which had a broken lock. She closed her own and said, 'Where's my draw? It's locked.' I readily concluded offering anything to Josephine was not going to be straightforward.

I suggested that she look at her toys and she took out some coloured bricks and started matching the colours, saying, 'Does green go with yellow?' etc. I pointed out that the colours she chose matched her dress and mine and said she might be wondering how well she and I would go with each other. She then became quite exuberant, built towers, and made them crash. I was talking about her worries in coming to see me – a strange person in a strange room, and how hard it was for her not to be in charge. She said, 'I think you are feeling worried about me coming to see you.'

We talked about the therapy being a place for *her* to come and play and talk about her worries, and she said, 'It's talking therapy,' a phrase which came back to us often in later sessions. She decided to paint and made some shapes – I had to guess whether they were a house or a car. Whichever I chose she then made into the opposite. I said she was putting me into the wrong each time – showing me *her* worry about getting things wrong; about being little and not being in control. I said I thought she felt that if she wasn't in control it would be dreadful – that everything would go wrong. In this first session, I thus learnt two of Josephine's main defences, her attempts to put all her worries into someone else and her need to control. As therapy progressed, I learnt poignantly of the things that had happened to her in reality when she lost this control. I saw her the next week, but the third week I had flu. I now quote some of her third session, which thus took place after a two-week gap. Josephine came quickly – dashed upstairs ahead of me – started to go the wrong way – running ahead and stumbled down small stairs, and I told her not to rush. In the room she ran to the drawers – closed her own drawer – opened the top one which is permanently unlocked, and said, looking at me jokingly, 'Where are my things? You threw them in the rubbish bin.' 'That was naughty of me,' I joked in return. She laughed, closed the drawer, and opened her own. I said she had worried that I hadn't looked after her things properly when I was away.

She said, 'I screamed every day when you weren't here,' demonstrated, and kicked me. I said something and she said, 'I hate you because you were away.' I said she was worried that the screaming and the angry feelings had kept me away, and that I wasn't there then to look after the screaming. She said, 'I thought you were dead.' We talked about this through the session. At times she seemed to be parroting me, at other times genuinely seeing if, for instance, my heart was still beating.

Later in the session, she played with plasticine and let me help her make two balls. She put them together to make a figure, said something about a tummy, then said, 'It split.' She had been talking about me being away, and about the holiday coming, and I said she was worried about my tummy being split and that it was her fault. She turned on me, kicking, screaming, and splitting. I talked about her worries about the time when I was ill – that it was her angry feelings with me that had made me ill. She meanwhile noticed the other set of drawers in the room and tugged at them. I said that she felt I had gone off with another baby in my tummy and she was angry about that. She went on spitting and screaming, and saying, 'What's frightened? What's worried?' 'You're frightened, you're worried,' and I said the spitting and screaming was to spit and scream out the frightened feelings, and that she kept thinking I was going to spit them back into her. She was also saying 'piss off' and 'fuck off' and asked if I would tell her Mummy. I said it was all private here and I wouldn't tell her Mummy or her teacher. She put eyes on the plasticine figure and then said, 'It's got eyes on its tummy.' I asked what she was thinking about eyes, and she said nothing. I said that when I had met her Mummy and Daddy they had told me she had had operations on her eyes. She said 'I haven't. I'm going to have one.' I said I thought she was telling me about her worries about the operation. We talked again of her worries that I was dead when I had flu because of what she had done to me, and what I might do to her, etc. She poked at my face and eyes as we talked.

She quietened down and started to do letters in her book. She told me about the children at home, adding one, an imagined brother Joseph, then naming herself and then her real brother. She went to the drawers again and we talked about her sharing her mother at home and me here, with the other children.

She wanted to take her plasticine figure home. I said she couldn't and she reminded me that I had let her take her paper model last week. 'You said "I'm not going to take it off you."' I said it had been a mistake to let her take it, and she said, 'You made a mistake so you've got to let me take this.' I said the mistake was in not keeping all the things together and all the feelings together – letting it spill outside the drawer and the room. She suddenly gave it back to me, then tried to trap my fingers in the drawer, and rushed out of the room and recklessly downstairs, but slowed down as she got to the classroom.

As you can see, she used therapy from the beginning, has been aware of the possibilities and the rules: she has known it was a 'talking therapy' and words, actions, and emotions have fumbled out. In that third session, the issue of privacy came up and was one of the themes of her therapy. She was apparently hurt when she discovered that I would not answer questions about myself, but it became a sort of ironical game – she would ask me a question and then mockingly say 'It's private,' which was not, I hasten to say, a quotation from me. The difficulty then was that if I asked her a question about home, her almost invariable answer was 'It's private.' I suspect however that this was useful as a formula and that it really was difficult for her to tell me in explicit terms about the dealings she had at home with her family. What she did not fail to communicate was the essence of it all in the transference. In fact, when she thought I might actually answer a question about myself she became very anxious.

In the school situation, she was very keen for me to preserve *her* privacy but could misuse her relationship with me cruelly towards other children. One needy little girl whose therapy elsewhere had had to stop, often said 'Hullo' to me. Josephine said to her 'Don't say hullo to my therapist. She's a stranger to you.' Another time, as she left the classroom to see me, she said meaningfully '*Therapy*, Jonathan' to a child whose therapist was away.

In that third session, we were able to see how she spits out and screams out the attacks she feels are going to happen to her. When I had been ill with flu it seemed she felt that my illness was due to her attacks on me and that the damaged me would attack *her*, and also be unable to protect her from attack.

Throughout the therapy Josephine has demonstrated that she feels constantly under attack – she is constantly expecting a 'smack in the face.' From her constantly provoking behaviour, it seemed likely that her expectations could easily be put into practice.

We have worked on her eye operation, both in preparation and afterwards. After the first one which took place during her time at the Day Unit, Josephine was able to spend a whole session acting out to me her experience, remembered and fantasised, of being on the operating table at the mercy of the surgeons, and of being blindfolded and helpless afterwards. In many subsequent sessions, she acted out a sadistic game in which she and I sat under a blanket in turns, and occasionally together. When I was under the blanket, she attacked me from outside and this seemed to be a way of communicating her experience in the dark in hospital. It again illustrated that Josephine's only defence is to project her fears into someone else. She is then terrified of the threat of it all being flung back at her. I hoped that my understanding of her fears would moderate this process and allow her to take it back in manageable doses.

Josephine's parents are unable to prepare her properly for traumatic events such as the eye operations, but I suspect that her extreme vulnerability precedes these betrayals and that they confirm rather than cause her feelings that she is always under threat. The nature of her disability – an eye defect – in itself was one of the causes of her vulnerability. Because she was literally unable to see clearly, she was unable to sift the dangers of her external world. At times, it must have seemed to her to be a jumble of persecution. When successive operations helped her to see more clearly, that in itself made her able to relate to the world with less anxiety.

Another theme was that of the birth of her younger brother, which came up in relation to other children in therapy with me. She probed my protection of her time, her toys, her privacy. She asked trick questions about whether I would allow her brother into the therapy room if she said it was alright and seemed satisfied with my absolute holding to the integrity of her therapy. She asked what would happen if he tried 'to smash his way in' and I talked about her feeling that he had smashed his way into Mummy's tummy and into their family and supplanted her as the baby. After this she talked, more distantly, of her elder sisters, and a hardly expressed but poignant feeling that she would never be the same as they were.

Josephine then moved up into an older age group at the beginning of the new school year. The next term was more difficult, with her screaming increasing. She often screamed at the beginning of a session, then had a quiet half-hour after getting solace from physical contact with me, or sucking her own thumb, and screaming again at the moment of re-entering the classroom. Talking beforehand about the pain of leaving therapy or of her destructive intent towards the children in the classroom did not alleviate this – the containment had to come from her teachers within the classroom.

The two last sessions before Christmas are of interest. In the first of these, she sobbed and kicked her way round the room, knocking over furniture and apparently not listening to what I said. In the next session she came in, quickly arranged two chairs touching and facing each other, and said, 'Lock my drawer, it's talking today.' She then took me through the sequence of the previous session, asking me to repeat my interpretations. 'What did you say when I kicked the table over?' We talked quietly and calmly of what I felt was her distress about the coming break, which seemed through her eyes to be endless – a black hole of desperation. It appeared to me that she had no surety that I or the Day Unit would be back for her after Christmas but also that it was not a simple experience of aloneness, or misery, but an active state of persecution in which she, alone, in the darkness, was going to be attacked. I also think that I, as the therapist, had been so attacked and damaged by her that I could not exist in her mind in my absence to convey her across such a break, and I then became one of her attackers. At that point I was not able to break into this dreadful sequence or convincingly see where it derived from; she conveyed it to me repeatedly without being able to get any relief from it.

At the time I wrote this last paragraph, Josephine's behaviour in the Unit as a whole was disruptive, and her spitting and screaming spoilt the classroom for the other children in the group. We had a meeting about her and I wrote this in preparation, conveying my doubts about her ability to use therapy. Following our meeting, the psychiatrist and teacher-in-charge spoke formally to Josephine's parents and to her. This had a most marked effect. She listened solemnly and made enormous efforts to curtail both the screaming and the spitting. I perhaps regretted that my interpretations had not alone been able to do this, but I appreciated the way in which the authority of the Day Unit was successful in setting limits for her. She then became able to differentiate her behaviour in therapy and in the rest of the Unit.

She continued to scream and spit in therapy, and I struggled to understand it in terms of her need to spit out and scream out the awful fears inside her. The arbitrary way in which her feelings of persecution could erupt were shown in two examples – when I had a bad cold she said in disgust, 'I will have to eat your snot,' and when I wore a pair of red boots with a zig-zag design she said, 'It's a crocodile. It's going to bite me.' Each time I wore them, the sight of the boots triggered off this response, although through repetition it became a joke. Both these instances show how vulnerable she feels to attack and one can sympathise with her parents in their lack of success in protecting her from the persecution of her operations. I think we can see how unusually vulnerable she is and how much more of a prey she is to such fantasies than are most children who undergo such experiences.

Her screaming and spitting subsided except for the unfortunate habit of screaming as she re-entered the classroom after the session. My interpretations became less sympathetic as I could see how she spoiled the quiet of the classroom. An identical grimace of pain and perhaps anger would pass over her teachers' faces and mine as the ear-splitting sound emerged. In fact, they then eased this enormously by being ready for her when she appeared. She was bundled into an armchair and held by one of the staff. The sympathy and containment *they* gave her at this moment in fact connected better with the experience she had had within the therapy room than did my own feeling towards her of betraying the resolution of her destructiveness, which we had each time achieved within the room. I was grateful to her teachers for the way they managed this period. Josephine betrayed the very privacy of her sessions which was so important to her when she spilled over in this way. I felt that her teachers made the empathic leap I described earlier, into knowing what she needed, without displaying undue curiosity, or undue criticism of my management of her.

By the next term, Josephine's parents had decided she would be better at boarding school and had discussed it with her. Josephine told me of this and scrutinised the expression on my face. She said, 'Is it a sad face or a happy face?' She wanted to know if I was happy to get rid of her, or sad to see her go. We discussed how she could say goodbye to the Unit and to me without spoiling all the good things we had had together and about how to remember someone inside you when you were no longer with them.

The next session she produced 2p from her dungaree pocket and said, 'That's for the therapy.' I said that she did not need to pay me for it, but I knew she was telling me she was grateful for what we had done together. She said with great meaning 'You said *talk*,' and I said I thought she was grateful for my helping her talk about things with words instead of screaming and kicking to show her feelings. She then rather spoilt our mood of self-congratulation by spitting in my face. When I protested she said, 'Miss B says I can spit in therapy because that's my problem,' a rather unconstructive reference back to the talk she had had with the psychiatrist and teacher incharge when she had learnt to differentiate her behaviour inside and outside therapy.

One area of protection of me is worth noting here. Throughout her attacking of me, she has always protected my handbag, and I have thought of this as being an extension of myself. Before overturning furniture, she carefully lifts my bag and puts it in a comer. In a recent session she said, 'I'll put your bag on that chair.' I said, 'thank you' and she said, 'I knew you'd say that.' I have never risked interpreting this split and spoiling the bag's special status but I think her acknowledgement of my thanks has meaning for her.

In recent sessions, she had told me obliquely of her masturbation which I felt was partly connected with her anger in bed at night at feeling excluded by me and by her parents. She continued some overtly sexual display – wanting to take off her knickers and finally in one session asked me to smack her (fully clothed) bottom. My interpretations did not divert her, and in order to further the work I joined in the game and pretended to smack her. The results were illuminating. She retaliated on me, and I said I thought she believed this was what mummies and daddies did in bed together and how they made babies. Then I said I thought she was trying to smack the babies out of Mummy's inside. Josephine was delighted with this remark and repeated it many times. The next session she began by chanting, 'Smack the baby out' and tried to reinstate the game. I was then inspired to say that I thought Josephine really wanted to be my baby and Mummy's baby, and have lots and lots of cuddles. She didn't know how to get me to give them to her, and at home she didn't know how to get Mummy to give them to her, so she tried to get smacked instead and was naughty until Mummy smacked her. Josephine said, 'How do you know about home?' and I said I didn't, I was working it out from what she told me. She came up close and spat straight in my face and I said I also thought spitting might be kissing – that she really wanted to be close and kiss people but she spat instead because she didn't know if they would want to kiss her. She became very clinging and got me to tuck her up in a blanket on the couch. She was very reluctant to leave and asked if she could marry me. I said how hard it was to leave me and the Day Unit when she went to her new school and she said, 'You can't marry ladies.' She got up quietly, got me to carry her down the corridor, and went quietly back to her classroom.

In another session, she again asked me to marry her but in a joking, 'refer-ring-back' way. Then she said she would like to have babies but not to get married, so she would find a good friend and ask him to make a baby with her. I asked her why she didn't want to get married, and she said she didn't want to sleep in the same bed as someone.

The poignancy is that it is very difficult to envisage this little girl as manag-ing marriage or parenthood. Although we could see her worry about marriage as an oedipal defence, it seems more likely that her enormous problems about separation are the key. She can only see herself as totally merged or totally separate. The end of a therapy session is so impossible to contemplate that she goes from being my baby in a blanket, wrapped in timeless care, to merg-ing infinitely with me in marriage. What she cannot be is a little girl walking separately down the corridor after her session. I think her repudiation of mar-riage is like her eliciting of smacks instead of cuddles, her spitting instead of kissing. She cannot stand a closeness that includes endings and separations so she forfeits the closeness.

Meanwhile, we are working on an ending, of her time in therapy, at the Day Unit, and at home. We have talked about how to take in and keep things good inside her, and she has told me that her teacher suggested taking photographs away with her. She worries that we are sending her off to a school that has the cane and has asked if the teachers there will be patient. She jokingly tells me that the teacher in charge has arranged for me to go with her to boarding school so that she can have therapy there. I find this quite a hopeful sign. She knows I will not go with her – but I think she is assuming my continued existence even if I do not. Both she and I are expected to survive the separation.

Josephine has improved noticeably in her behaviour at the Unit. She is much more contained, she looks more mature, is sometimes thoughtful towards the other children, and her learning has increased rapidly. At home, she is more manageable but boarding school is still the realistic place for her because there is no suitable day school. She provides a good example of someone for whom neither therapy nor the therapeutic environment separately could have effected the change that the two together have achieved. The constant repeti-tion of interpretations about her anxieties while being held in an environment that was both understanding and also authoritative where necessary somehow helped her constant experience of persecution to diminish. This abated and she was able to take in more and more what we could offer her and to substitute expected good experiences for some of the bad ones. Her thoughts about boarding school show that she still projects her own sadistic impulses into the unknown, the teachers who will cane her, but our hope is that if the teachers there are really, in her words, 'patient,' that is, if they can manage to contain the jumble of her anxieties and make sense of them, she will again be able to internalise real good experiences. Our hope is that she will be able to link her use of all of us at the Day Unit with this future experience.

Reference

Daws, D. (1977) 'Child Psychotherapy in a Day Unit' in Ed. Daws, D. & Boston, M. *The Child Psychotherapist and the Problems of Young People*. London: Routledge.

Part 4
Writing for parents

10 The one-year-old and his family

Originally a chapter from Your One Year Old *(1969).*

Parents

The independence of your one-year-old is really only relative. In spite of his forays into the grownup world, your one-year-old is hardly more than a baby himself. In the course of a long day spent practising new skills, and exercising his rights to freedom, he may many times subside into a helpless bundle sucking his thumb. His existence on two such extreme levels is what in turn delights and exhausts his mother. She must keep up with his need to have the boundaries of his world pushed farther and farther away and still remain available as the loving encompassing mother of his infancy.

The one-year-old is learning to move away from his mother: when he crawls it is away from her, to the intriguing other side of the room, to the wonders outside the door. When he walks, his speed and range of movement increase again and the whole house or flat is his for the taking. But the more he goes away from his mother's side, the more he must be sure she is there to come back to, and that she is not having thoughts of going away herself. In fact, the more he stretches his own limits of confidence and daring, the more he needs to be able to retreat back to her side.

His very confidence in himself is rooted in his relationship with his mother and later with his father. Through his first year, this relationship has developed and with it have come feelings about himself. As he develops, they become increasingly incorporated, and later when he grows up he will carry these inner feelings along with him wherever he goes. If the relationship with the mother has been one of acceptance by her, he will have a sense of inner security and confidence. On the other hand, if the relationship is marked by uneasiness or tension he may not be able to build up a picture of himself as an integrated person, and may never attain the ability to deal successfully with the world. In

DOI: 10.4324/b23125-14

any case now, he has to continue to refer back to his mother as the source of these feelings.

His sorties out into the world followed by a quick scuttle back to mother's side are pretty easy to take. What are much more difficult for the mother are the long periods of new discovery when the baby stretches his nerves to the limits, followed by perhaps longer ones where he seems to go to pieces and for a while becomes a clinging little creature quite unable to let his mother out of his sight. He trails around after her all day, not able even to let her go the lavatory alone, and screams if he is left alone briefly outside a shop. This is the picture of a baby who has, for the moment, over-reached himself. His self-confidence took him too far, and he is telling his mother he did not really mean it and that suddenly he feels he is a little baby again who should not be left for a moment. He is in fact frightened at the degree of independence he has achieved for himself and that has been accorded him within the family. For the moment he is retrenching, but any day now he will be bursting out of these self-imposed limits again.

So far, I have really only described one kind of baby, the kind who bursts into his second year of life with a strong demand for freedom. Others may ease themselves into this stage so gently that any problems hardly seem to show. Some self-possessed children seem able to regulate their rate of development to a pace with which they can cope, and the periods of insecurity or frustration are few.

Mothers differ too in their reaction to their child striking out for himself. Some are conservative and slow to adapt to changing needs. Some have so much enjoyed the experience of cherishing an infant that they are very reluctant to give this up. They resent their baby no longer needing them so totally. Yet another kind of mother is uneasy in the intimate bodily contact of the first year and comes into her own in the kind of relationship demanded by the more independent child. She may have few difficulties in allowing him increasing freedom, and she will encounter fewer problems at this stage.

Some mothers and babies have a difficult first year together. The baby always seems to be crying for inexplicable reasons, and the mother often feels herself anxious as new stages bring still more problems. Sometimes, to a mother and baby in this situation, the coming of the second year brings a release. The baby suddenly seems to settle down, and the mother finds herself well able to cope.

What now of our baby's father? I have talked first of the mother because the relationship with her is the first important one in the baby's life. She has carried him in her body, given birth to him, and may actually have provided him with his first food from her own body, so that the physical link between them is not broken for a while. From this intimate bodily contact, a loving relationship builds up between a mother and her baby.

Although the father cannot share directly in this physical relationship, it is still vital for him to be there. Not only can he support the mother emotionally, and keep the world away from her in the weeks of her being absorbed in the baby, but also he can share in the loving feelings, the wonder and the fears of having a small human being entrusted to one. In the last few years, fathers have been encouraged to participate in their wives' pregnancies, and they may often be fortunate enough to see their own baby being born so that they are able to experience the excitement of birth and to know their baby from its first moment of life.

To these fathers, there is usually no difficulty in making contact with their baby, and the relationship builds up gradually through the first year. Other fathers may find this first stage more difficult, feeling it is a period that belongs to the mother and baby alone and that they themselves are a little excluded. However, the importance of all fathers to the baby is shown unmistakably after the first few months. The radiant smile a father can get simply by walking into a room is well known as a source of delight and exasperation to the mother who works all day tending her baby. But it is precisely the difference in the roles of mother and father which is so important.

The relationship to mother at first is a life and death one, and mother and baby experience emotions of frightening intensity. The mother is rewarded with the baby's first smiles and feels these as a recognition of herself by her baby. When the baby's world enlarges to include his father, a different quality can often be seen in the smiles and special sounds he saves for him. From very early on, this difference in the way the baby treats each parent can be seen, and often the father is used as a means of escape from the intense link between the baby and his mother. The emotions between mother and baby are intense and often painful. The baby is dependent on his mother in every way, and as well as loving he may often feel angry with her. The strength of his own emotions frightens him. It can therefore be a relief to get away from these to his father, who is still extremely important to him but without this basic painfulness.

By the time our baby is one year old, the difference in relation to each parent is still very much there, though many more elements are now added. Father is still the very special person whose every appearance is heralded with excitement. In most families, father goes out to work and comes back regularly so that he disappears and appears again. His reappearance then is a special event. Mother, on the other hand, is nearly always there, and is expected to be there, caring for the baby.

In his relation to the father, the baby learns that there is a world outside the home. He learns to be able to say goodbye, to remember his father in his absence during the day, and to anticipate his return at bedtime. There may well be tears when father says goodbye in the morning but then the baby can settle down into the daily routine with his mother, knowing father will come back. Many small children will play with something belonging to their father at intervals during the day perhaps to assure themselves of his return. At 15 months when his father got up out of his chair, Keith would mischievously climb into it. You could almost see him thinking, 'I'm Daddy now.' During the day when father was at work, Keith would often sit in the chair for a few moments. always with the same air that this was somewhere privileged to be. While he was there he had father's presence around him.

The constant relationship with mother is bound up in the daily intimate routine of caring for the baby and responding to its needs. But in doing this, mother can become rather conservatively bound up with the baby as he is at a given moment. By contrast, father coming fresh into the situation, may well be the initiator of little games that help stretch the baby's capabilities. He may be able to point out to mother that the baby has reached some new stage that she has not allowed herself to recognise and is perhaps curbing. As someone concerned, but not directly involved, he can often help to break the deadlock between mother and baby which this sort of situation brings about. When, for instance, feeding difficulties become severe and tension has built up between mother and baby, father may be able to step in and release them from their conflict with each other.

As well as relating to his mother and father as two separate people, our one-year-old begins to comprehend them as a married couple. Sometimes, we have the feeling that he would like to keep them as two separate people. Somehow he is always getting in between them. He turns up in the night and climbs into bed between his parents. In the daytime when they are talking to each other, he will break into the conversation. Sometimes, when he seems to be trying to keep his parents apart we feel his envy of this relationship which excludes him. At other times, he may be asking to be included in the loving relationship he can see before him. When his parents kiss each other, he will want them to kiss him too so that he can share in their affection without spoiling it, and we can see how important the strength of the bond between his parents is for the child.

Now that the baby responds to both mother and father, sexual differences in the attitude towards them often shows. In some families, little girls are noticeably more cuddly with their fathers, while little boys may be more demonstrative with their mothers.

At 18 months, Ann would openly flirt with her father across the table, catching his eye, looking coyly away, and turning back to smile at him. At 16 months Peter enjoyed exciting games with his father, but when he sat in his high chair he would lovingly draw his mother towards him so that her cheek would rest on his. However, both boys and girls seem to need mother most when they are not well or when waking up in the night either with teething pains or nightmares. At these times, their pain or fears take them back to being babies again, to the time when mother was their sole source of comfort.

Father's approval or disapproval is often felt much more strongly than mother's. A baby will try his hardest to dazzle father with his new tricks and be delirious with excitement when father responds to him. On the other hand, father's displeasure really seems to strike at the roots of his self-esteem. A mild telling-off that might brush over his head if it came from mother can reduce him to tears when it comes from father.

The difference in relation to mother and father could be seen in Daniel's attitude to his parents' absence when he was 13 months old. His mother, who had never left him before, went away overnight with father, leaving Daniel with grandmother, whom he knew well. When mother the day, Daniel was sitting on grandmother's lap happily playing. For ten minutes, he gave no sign of having noticed mother, then he warily allowed her to take hold of him, gradually warming to her as she talked to him. However, when father returned three days later, having continued on a business trip, Daniel's immediate reaction was to rush over to him shouting ecstatically, 'Dadda, Dadda.' The moral is clear. Daniel had been able to manage fairly happily without mother while she was away, but when she came back he had to express his feeling that mothers should not really go away. They should be there all the time, and if they went away they became strangers. His feeling towards father, however, did not depend on his continual presence, and while father was away he did not have to develop this rift between them. Father could both go away and come back more easily than could mother.

Brothers and sisters

The one-year-old who is the first or only child enjoys a special relationship with his parents. He has their love and attention all for himself without having to share it with other children in the family. Younger children never experience this, having the parents all to themselves, from the beginning they must compete with their brothers and sisters. What they gain is in being at once a member of a family, of having a part in its network of relationships.

He spends much of his time watching, admiring, and envying his older brothers and sisters. How he gets on with them depends, of course, on the personalities of all the children concerned, but one important variable is the age-gap.

Keith, whose two older brothers were, respectively, seven and five years older than him, found himself in a very favoured position in the family. Both older brothers, who had experienced considerable rivalry and jealousy between themselves at a younger age, went out of their way to be nice to Keith. They spent long periods playing games carefully geared to his abilities and were generally loving and protective towards him. When Keith was cross at bedtime, his oldest brother could put him to bed when no one else could. The only time this brother was really angry with Keith and shouted at him was when Keith tore a favourite book of his. Keith was very frightened at this unaccustomed anger, and his brother was conscience stricken.

The one-year-old with brothers and sisters nearer to his own age will get a different picture of what the world is like. He may already as a tiny baby have had to be protected by his mother from the jealous attacks of his older siblings. He may have been 'loved' in a too hearty manner. He will already be learning in the light of his own personality to withstand all this. What he will have gained is the stimulus of having an older child around. Moreover, a child can be violently jealous of his younger brother or sister at one moment and genuinely delight in some accomplishment at the next. Perhaps through the baby he can relive some of the happy moments of his own babyhood. The baby born into a family that already has children has a very different environment from the first-born or only child whose early contacts are mainly with its mother and father, adults whose emotions are kept in a moderate degree of control. The child born later in the family comes into contact with all the excesses of the other children's behaviour. Sometimes it is helpful to see other children only at a stage more civilised than oneself. Sometimes it can be worrying to the baby to witness the strong feelings of an older child or to see him punished. Keith looked frightened whenever mother shouted at the older boys or when the dog was smacked.

Older children can be a very helpful spur to development for a younger one. Parents can often seem to be so proficient and their achievements unattainable. It is much more realistic to compare oneself with a big brother or sister where the gap in ability is not so wide.

The one-year-old is in a particularly vulnerable position as far as jealousy from an older one is concerned. Although an older child may be acutely jealous of a baby's very existence and of the mother's care of it, the baby does stay in its own special infant world and can be forgotten at times. But a one-year-old cannot be ignored, he actually intrudes into the older child's world. Instead of lying helplessly in his cot, he crawls and walks, he toddles into the very place where the older one is playing and upsets his games. He rivals the older one with his new skills in manipulating toys. When Mark was given a wooden post-box for his first birthday, he quickly learned to fit the simpler pieces into the holes. At first, his older brother could not bear to see him do this. He would snatch the toy away and condescendingly show Mark how to post all the pieces. Then he managed to restrain his feelings sufficiently to allow Mark to play with it, but the game had to be under his control. He selected the pieces for Mark, and as the baby fitted each piece through the correct hole, his brother shouted patronisingly, 'Clever boy.' In a family comprising more than a mother and father, the child creates a wider circle of relationships. It can be a great strain for an only child to have to focus the full intensity of all his emotions on to the relationships between himself and his two parents. An only child, or one who has not yet got younger brothers or sisters, needs a few close companions to allow him some freedom in using different people as recipients of different emotions at some difficult moments in life. Grandparents can fulfil a particularly valuable role in this respect. When emotions towards the parents are painfully intense, escape to the grandparents can be a great relief. At other times, the child may use one parent as an escape from the other.

During this year, the child's mother may well become pregnant again. The child will feel his mother as being absorbed in something else, as having less time for him, less room for him on her lap. He is in fact ousted by the newcomer well before its birth. The child, however young, can be greatly helped through all his feelings about this, his jealousy, his despair at being displaced by another baby, by his parents talking to him about it, and allowing him to express these feelings in words and in actions. By accepting the violence and the fluctuating nature of these feelings, they allow him to work through them at his own pace. Putting all this into words enables the child to feel that all these parts of him have been accepted by the parents – he feels understood and loved by them.

11 Love and hate

Originally a chapter from **Your One Year Old** *(1969).*

The baby's strongest feelings are still those towards his mother and father, and as well as loving feelings, he has equally strong hating feelings. When mother stops her one-year-old from doing something he wants to do, the strength of his fury can be amazing to see.

With Peter we saw a small outburst when his mother stopped him climbing on her and grabbing the scissors. He resolved this by throwing the bricks about. Another child might directly hit his mother, and this could also be a way of showing his feelings and quickly dispelling them. However, as this year progresses, it seems to become more and more difficult to get rid of the anger in this easy and direct way, and the child's anger becomes choked up in a temper tantrum.

Temper tantrums are a mixture of frustration and anger which become so violent that the child is completely overwhelmed, and often he seems powerless to stop them. He needs his mother, towards whom his feelings are directed at depth, to step in and help him. He often needs her to hold him physically so that the feelings that are spilling over everywhere are held in check for him. When these tantrums happen outside the home, as often embarrassingly seems to be the case, it may relieve the situation if the mother removes the child bodily from the place where the frustration occurred and then talks quietly and calmly about whatever sparked off the tantrum.

When a child gets into this state, he becomes terrified himself by his own violence, and he fears it may destroy himself and his mother. When the mother strongly but lovingly holds her child, he may continue to scream, but she will feel him listening as she talks calmly to him. Even a 20-month-old can respond when his mother shows that she respects the importance of whatever has caused his outburst and that she is able to hold him physically and emotionally through his anger, and not be upset or damaged by the violence of it.

DOI: 10.4324/b23125-15

After he has begun to listen to his mother, he will soon quieten down and will be able to talk in his simple vocabulary about what has happened. The holding by his mother represents a sort of holding together when he feels he is almost falling apart from the violence of his emotions. When he has been restored to a whole, then the holding provides the safe, loving background for mutual understanding on the much more mature level of words.

At other times, a child may need to be left to himself for a while during a tantrum. He may need the freedom to express the extreme emotions he is experiencing inwardly in the outward form of screaming, hurling himself on the floor, and kicking. Some children need to do this away from their mothers so that they are not afraid that the violence will harm her. They will then be able to recover spontaneously and come back lovingly to mother. The mother will then need to hold her baby so that he can feel that both the violent and the loving part of him has been reunited with an understanding mother.

Throughout this year, the mother tries to instil some sense of discipline within the child. She tries to set the limits of what the child may or may not do, and the child tests out these limits continually. At first, the child has no feeling within himself of right or wrong, of what is acceptable or unacceptable to his mother. He desists from forbidden behaviour solely in reference to his mother, and usually only when she is actually in the room reminding him. But although he sometimes seems very slow to learn the 'rules' of his home, progress does get made.

When Mark was 11 months old and his mother said 'No' as he touched electric plugs he just looked at her and laughed. At 12 months he looked at her, shook his head in agreement, and said 'No' before turning back to the plug. His mother optimistically felt some progress had been made in his appreciation of the situation. On the other hand, at 12 months Carol took it seriously when her mother said 'No' and would turn her head and stop what she was doing. At 15 months, however, when her mother shouted 'No,' Carol would come over, looking cross, and hit her.

At times like these, the mother can distract the baby with something else, either giving him another toy immediately or removing him quickly to the other side of the room, then presenting the alternative toy. Distracting a baby really does work if action is taken quickly before a big issue has built up. It has to be done tactfully – holding out the alternative before taking the forbidden object away. It is not, however, a short-cut; it will have to be done over and over again – but it can prevent the dreadful deadlock where a mother is saying 'No' and her baby just isn't taking any notice. At 23 months, Paul's mother often still had to distract him when he wanted to do something forbidden. As she put it, if she didn't take the trouble to distract him, she was leaving him high and dry with his aggressive feelings.

Valuable as this method can be, particularly at the beginning of this year, later on it should not become a substitute for allowing the child to really work through situations of frustration and cope with his feelings about it. As the year develops, the conflicts between parents and child must often be experienced, not evaded, if the child is to take into himself any feeling of what he may or may not do. The parent has to allow the child really to face the feelings of these confrontations before helping him through them.

It is now that mothers sometimes resort to smacking, and then feel guilty about it. Smacking probably does no more good than a serious tone of voice. It really acts as an expression of the mother's own temporary loss of temper, and a baby is quite capable of affectionately understanding it as such. If a mother often finds herself slapping her child, then something has gone wrong between herself and the child, and she needs to sit down quietly and revaluate the situation. Often what are needed at the age we are talking about are more safety precautions in the house, so that fewer battles of will between mother and baby are stirred up.[1]

Babies vary tremendously in the robustness with which they can take an admonition from their parents. Where one may be quite unmoved by a grave tone of voice, another will burst into tears, afraid that the parents' sternness means they no longer love him. The same child may react in totally different ways at different stages of this year. At 16 months Keith, who might have been quite unmoved or smilingly defiant earlier on in the year, took his mother's purse. She took it away from him and offered him a toy in exchange. He brushed this away, dissolved into tears and put his arms around mother's neck. He then did allow her to take him over to the window, where he looked out with interest then happily switched a light on and off. Suddenly, he remembered his grief and cried again. Mother put him on father's special chair. From here he climbed proudly onto the table but suddenly cried again. Mother unconcernedly went out, and he climbed down, toddled after her, found a push toy and happily wheeled it along.

In this incident, we see Keith's grief not only at losing the purse he wants but also at feeling that mother is disapproving of him. He bursts into tears and puts his arms around her to win her back. She comforts him by holding him, and he can then let himself be distracted by his favourite activities of looking out of the window and turning on the light. When he continues to complain, she does not let the situation drag on, but by casually going about her own work, allows the tension between them to drop.

Carol, at 15 months, had been waking a great deal at night. One night she had been crying noisily, and mother had gone into her several times. Finally, mother went in and said angrily to Carol that she was keeping everyone awake. Carol was quiet at once. In a very small voice, she said, 'Mummy.' She sounded stricken at the anger her own crying had evoked.

Paul who had been a happy, easy child became aggressive at 23 months. He would frequently bite his parents or brothers. His mother connected this biting with the fact that he was cutting four back teeth. She felt perhaps that he was trying to get rid of the biting pain inside his own mouth by biting his family. When he bit anyone, he was usually smacked by mother; his aggression would then disappear at once and he would cry. He would then want to make it up with mother and hold his arms out to her and she would pick him up and cuddle him.

With Paul again we see how punishment feels like a loss of mother's love – his aggression goes and he must win her back at once.

At 23 months Daniel became unable to tolerate the guilt aroused when his parents were cross with him. He would hit his head and say very pathetically, 'Bump me.' They were then supposed to be very sorry for him – stop being cross and kiss him better. If this didn't work with one parent, he would 'bump' himself still harder and go off to complain louder to the other parent. This was his way of dominating his feelings of guilt by attempting to change the situation around to suit his needs and so have control over his parents' reactions to him.

Sometimes a small child will be able to cope with the parents' mild crossness towards himself but become very anxious when older children are spoken to sternly or perhaps smacked. When Carol was told off herself she showed little reaction, but when she heard her older brother crying in the next room she would worry until she went to see what was the matter with him.

In another situation Jenny, aged 20 months, was sitting near mother, who was breast-feeding James, then five months old. We have already met poor Jenny's difficulties and jealousy of her brother at feeding time. Jenny sat swinging her legs and kicked mother, at first accidentally, then on purpose. Mother told her to stop, at first with no effect, but when she repeated it more severely Jenny burst into tears, and was only comforted when mother told her she hadn't been *very* naughty. Jenny then exuberantly spread herself over mother's lap, half covering the baby who was sitting up to wind. He looked uncomfortable and put his hand over Jenny's knee. Mother told Jenny to move and said she could sit on her knee. Jenny sat on the outside of mother's knee with the baby near to mother. After a moment, she slid off and played in the next room. Jealousy as displayed by Jenny towards James is one of the most painful of human emotions. We have already seen how it led to nightmares and sleeplessness for Jenny. But we mustn't overlook the positive aspect of jealousy – for instance, a child who is jealous of sharing his parents with a younger brother or sister is showing how much he values a relationship he is reluctant to share.

Jealousy can also be a spur to development, often amusingly so; Carol at 15 months found her mother and three-year-old brother doing exercises. She couldn't bear not to join in. She made mother lie down, pushed herself against mother's chest and stood up for the very first time. When everyone clapped and she was once more the centre of attention, she beamed with delight.

Daniel aged 22 months had always been charmingly paternal to a neighbour's child now aged 12 months so long as she remained a baby crawling about on the floor. Things changed as she began to grow up. One day she pulled herself up by the coffee-table and stood. Daniel took one look at her and climbed *on to* the table. Honour was restored.

The very mixed feelings a baby has towards its parents, especially mother, in times of stress is shown in his behaviour when he is hurt. Many babies when they are hurt will come to mother to be comforted but then stiffen as she picks them up and hold themselves away from her as they cry. This is because, although the baby is learning so much about the world, and probably hurt himself while exploring it, he still often feels that everything that happens to him good or bad is really caused by his mother. Although he is beginning to see himself in relation to an external world, a crisis such as being hurt sends him back to this earlier stage, and he feels that his pain must be his mother's fault; in fact, she must have hurt him.

When Daniel, at 14 months, was playing with a heavy tin and dropped it on his toe he screamed and flung himself away from his mother, who was trying to pick him up to comfort him. Not till the pain had subsided a little, and with it his panic, could he turn to his mother, who had for a short time been a fearful person who hurt babies.

Thumb-sucking is one of the ways in which a baby comforts himself by means of part of his own body. Thus, he need not be dependent on his mother for all his comfort – it is his solace when he must be on his own. Normally this is a healthy way of dealing with loneliness, sadness, or sleepiness. Carol's mother commented that Carol, who sucked her thumb, was happier and easier to deal with than her older brother and sister, who had never sucked theirs. When Mark at 12 months was sleepy, he would suck his left thumb and pull his ear. Together with his far-away dreamy expression, this gave him an air of being comfortably sufficient unto himself. However, he could easily return to contact with his mother. If she picked him up when he was in this state, he would smile and snuggle up against her. Only if a baby continually sucks his thumb or fingers with disturbing intensity and still looks anxious – not seeming to get the comfort he is seeking – or if when he sucks he becomes so withdrawn that this state seems more important and real to him than contact with people – should we feel there is cause to worry and seek expert help.

Similarly, in times of distress some masturbation and rocking can be a normal quest for comfort from the baby's own body. But again if the masturbation or rocking are continued and violent we might guess that this is a baby who is unable to show his angry or aggressive feelings directly at the time they are aroused. A baby like this may sometimes feel very angry towards his parents but is so afraid of the strength of this anger that he cannot express it. He is still at the stage where he cannot distinguish feelings from actions. His feelings seem so powerful that sometimes he fears they may actually harm his parents, whom he needs and loves, or sometimes he fears that such strong anger must call up equally strong anger in them. Either way, these feelings are too dangerous to express towards them, and the alternative he finds is to turn the feelings on to his own body – expressing them in an angry kind of masturbation, rocking, or head-banging. A baby who is doing this violently is unhappy and needs help.

Note

1 This was written in 1969 and is now out of date, with smacking no longer seen as an acceptable practice. I was working with the practices that took place within families at the time.

12 Crying babies

Originally a chapter from Finding Your Way With Your Baby *(2015), co-written with* *Alexandra de Rementeria.*

Listening and comforting

All babies cry. They cannot yet talk, so crying is a way to communicate their feelings. Some babies do cry more than others, but when a new baby cries, there is always a reason: they are not trying to manipulate you, they do need you for something.

A newborn's cry is almost irresistible. It pulls adults towards the baby, often without them consciously noticing they have responded.

From parents . . .

When a friend visited with her three-week-old baby, I found myself half-way up the stairs as the baby gave her first cry, before remembering she wasn't mine – even though my own children were long grown up by then!

Why babies cry

Crying is instinctive: its purpose is to bring an adult close to keep the baby alive, by feeding and keeping her safe. There are several main causes of crying, such as hunger, pain, discomfort, loneliness, or overstimulation. Your baby will probably develop a number of different cries and in time you will be able to differentiate these, although you may not be aware that you are doing it.

Babies are not always in distress when they cry. At these times the cry will not be upsetting to listen to, nor will it be an ordeal to sort out what the baby wants. In fact, hearing the sounds your baby makes can be part of the amazing discovery of this new little person. The cry of a baby a few weeks old can have a musical lilt that is very pleasant to hear. By crying, your baby not only

DOI: 10.4324/b23125-16

lets you know that she's hungry or tired or that she just needs some attention; she also wants to sense your nearness and feel safe. Your response to her cries shows her that you are available and helps to strengthen the feeling that she can depend on you. Babies do not always know themselves why they are crying – they may have a general feeling of misery or of just needing 'something' and need you to understand this. Giving them attention may then be sufficient in itself to satisfy them.

Many babies have a 'crying period' at a certain time daily that doesn't appear to be related to hunger or any of the usual causes. This 'unexplained crying' often happens in the evening when you are also at your most tired. Fortunately, it is often followed by your baby's longest sleep period, so you all have a chance to recover. It is also helpful to think that babies who cry a lot are being assertive and that this is a very positive character trait. They are able to let their parents know about discomfort or dissatisfaction. Some 'good' babies, who rarely cry, may not be able to assert their own wishes so effectively. Ill babies must, of course, never be left to cry – your doctor or health visitor can help you to differentiate the sound of a sick baby's cry if you are not confident that you will know this yourself.

Comforting your baby

Babies are usually very ready to be soothed. They will stop crying as soon as an adult picks them up, either because they enjoy being held or because they can anticipate that their need is about to be met. A baby of only a few days will stop crying at the sound of her mother's voice, apparently knowing that she is there and is coming for her. This is also one of a baby's first experiences of cause and effect. Soon a baby will start to pause between bouts of crying to listen to whether someone is coming.

From parents . . .

Getting ready to go out with a newborn was hard. Having put him in the buggy I would be hurriedly going to the loo, getting my coat on and so on, all the while chatting to my baby boy because he would cry at our physical separation. At about three weeks old, I noticed that he would, for a little while, stop his crying to listen, clearly paying attention to (and comforted by) the sound of my voice. I, in turn, found this decidedly reassuring.

From research on the biochemistry of cuddling . . .

Schore (2001) described research showing that when a distressed infant is held ventral to ventral (chest to chest), heart rate matching occurs, which resets the baby's autonomic nervous system. The mother's autonomic nervous system thus acts directly on that of the baby, bringing it back to normal. This not only calms the baby in that moment but the mother's body is 'training' the baby's body to adjust the balance of adrenaline and noradrenaline in his system in order to bring it back to normal.

Learning to recognise the meaning of your baby's cries is one of the main ways that you get to know each other. In fact, most babies will react to whatever their parents try. At first, babies will need to feed or, at least suck, when they cry. But they may also simply enjoy bodily contact with their mother or father. Holding your baby close to you, chest to chest, is one of the most successful positions to soothe a baby: it lets her know that you are emotionally open to her. The physical proximity enables you to feel her distress, and she in turn can feel, through your body, your wish to know about her feelings and to comfort her. Some babies like to be held higher, against your shoulder.

Talking to your baby, rather than just holding her silently, is also important. Provided that you are not feeling too upset yourself, your voice can echo some of the lilt of her cry as you ask her how she is, with something like 'Poor Baby. What's the matter?' Having become in tune with her emotions like that, you may find yourself calmly telling her 'It's alright, Mummy's here.'

The fussy or inconsolable baby

Each baby requires a unique approach from her parents. Some babies seem to be born more fussy or irritable than others. They cry more than their siblings or peers, which may demand sensitive thinking about how to help them. If she goes on crying after you have been through all the usual checks of whether she is in pain, hungry, or wet, it could be that it is simply taking her a while to settle down after her birth. The world is a very different place from the womb!

If the birth was difficult, she may have had a jangled start and you may have to work harder than usual to find ways of soothing her. All babies have their own preferences for sounds, rhythms, and ways of being held. You may even have detected some of these personal preferences while she was still inside you – such as her reaction to music or a particular noise.

From parents ...

My firstborn cried a lot and really loud. I only started to realise that not all babies were like her when I went to a breastfeeding meeting. She had slept through it but woke as people got up to leave. Everybody stopped and stared in stunned silence at her blood-curdling scream. I was taken aback by their response. That was just the sound of her waking up. My son was completely different. His cry was a quiet mewing; at first I thought he was just talking to himself and didn't realise he was asking me for something.

When she would cry inconsolably and heartbreakingly and I couldn't calm her I felt so bad, so worried and then at times angry. I wish I could have known then that she would always have this thing where she would get on to an emotional trajectory and not be able to divert from it. Once she is mad, she stays mad until she's done and then she's fine. I wish I'd understood that my job was to bear it with her, be there while she did her thing, not necessarily to make it stop.

A baby who is crying may be communicating intense and passionate feelings of all kinds but especially of misery or anger. These are normal kinds of emotions, but when a mother or father, perhaps because of their own experiences, is frightened of what their baby is expressing, they will not be able to reassure her. She will be left unsettled, perhaps still crying, unable to sleep. If a parent can understand these feelings and help the baby to deal with them, repeated instances lead her to remember this and learn how to manage them herself. By trying to soothe your child, you demonstrate to her that you are doing your best to understand why she is crying and that you do have the resources to help her feel better.

Coping with prolonged crying

Soothing a crying baby is partly trial and error. The trouble is that you are not a dispassionate scientist doing an experiment in a quiet laboratory. The crying can get to you – get into you – while you are trying to figure out how to respond. As described earlier, babies cannot regulate their own autonomic nervous system; they do need another body to hold them close and do that for them. However, that other body, your body, may be that of a sleep-deprived and neurochemically chaotic person. You may be struggling with your own capacity to downregulate in a way that throws you back into being like a helpless raging baby again yourself.

From psychoanalytic theory and clinical practice . . .

It is often during a bout of prolonged crying that a mother is confronted by her own ambivalence, just at the moment when your baby most needs you to be available to her. One mother told me that her baby's crying made her so angry that she had to keep silent, or 'the things I would say to him would be too awful.' In fact, it wasn't until she was able to talk to me about these 'awful' thoughts of hostility towards her baby, and have them understood, that she was able to convincingly calm him when he cried.

From parents . . .

When she gets like that it feels quite crazy. I struggle to be the calm one because as much as she gets lost in that feeling, so can I. It's like she pulls me in with her.

Sometimes I had to speak of love when I was feeling hate and in time we both started to believe in, or remember, the fact that I do love her and we would both calm down. Other times I had to ask someone else to take her for a short while.

When your baby has gotten herself into a state and doesn't know how to get out of it unaided, if you can just bear her feelings with her you may be able to lessen their force and prevent either her or you from becoming too distraught. If your body or voice are shaking with suppressed hostility, you will make her feel frightened. If you are feeling very angry, you need the help of somebody else. This could be the other parent, a friend, or professional. They are not trying to take her from you but to help you both sort it out. It can be helpful to think about it in terms of your deserving support because what you are doing is important and difficult, not because you are no good at it.

From parents . . .

When I've been up for hours with her crying and arching away and I'm physically and mentally exhausted by the work of feeling those desperate feelings with her and the effort of trying to keep a lid on my building anger, I do resent the lack of status this work has. If I were doing some other job that demanded such self-sacrifice and exposure to raw emotions, it would be well paid and I'd have back up – not a lonely sense of doubt and failure.

We know about neuronal rewiring during the third trimester, which primes mothers to be more alert to danger, but it is one of evolution's worst snags because it actually makes us stressed and jumpy, just when we need to be calm for the baby. If we think of a mother, woken *again* in the night by screaming, we can picture her stumbling to the cot and picking the baby up – but he arches against her and screams harder. We feel the rage rip through her as her 'fight' response to stress is activated. Heroically, she will not act on this but instead she is left holding him with arms and neck rigid, heart racing, and an expression on her face that is somewhere between bewilderment and rage. She is trying to ignore what her body is telling her because she knows he needs her to comfort and soothe him and that is what she wants to do. However, he can only know her mind through his experience of her body, and her body is telling him that there is danger around. Boutaleb (2019) urged mothers to take a moment to notice this. Our hypothetical mother realises that her shoulders are up at her ears; she takes a deep breath and lets them drop. She takes a couple more slow, deep breaths, and this brings her heart rate down and allows her face to relax.

She has begun to regulate her own autonomic nervous system and now her baby begins to trust that she can help him to regulate his. He is right!

'Ghosts in the nursery'

We know that all parents can experience feelings of hostility towards their baby, but some will struggle with this more than others, especially when their baby is crying.

If your mother was rejecting, you may find that turning away or becoming angry are the only responses you know to the sound of a crying baby. The feelings that you had, that you were no good, when your mother seemed to be pushing you away get stirred up again. You feel rejected by your baby and reject her in return. However, it can be the very fact of being rejected that makes babies 'go on and on' crying. Babies can actually make do with and be satisfied with quite a small amount of comfort, but it can be hard to discover this if you don't feel that you have what they need. You can feel that your crying baby is telling you that you are no good, and this in turn makes you want to just shut her up. Parents who batter their babies often feel that the baby is criticising them when she cries. (An amazing 80% of parents with new babies said they could sympathise with people who batter their babies. This shows vividly how testing a crying baby can be.)

However, you need not have experienced neglect or abuse to find yourself grappling with 'ghosts in the nursery.' Many aspects of the way you parent will be influenced by the way you were parented in ways that it can be hard to bring into conscious awareness.

From psychoanalytic theory and clinical practice . . .

Sometimes parents are unable to soothe their babies because of something in their own history. Fraiberg et al. (1980) used the phrase 'ghosts in the nursery' to describe how problems between a parent and baby can often be traced back to the parent's experiences in infancy. Often, if people were neglected when they were themselves babies and their cries went unheard, their baby's crying stirs up their own unmet infantile needs and actually makes them feel unable to muster sufficient adult resources for their baby. It usually takes someone listening to their memories of childhood to help them get in control of these unmet needs. If parents are listened to, they will then most likely be able to listen to their baby's cries and console them.

In the terrible (and thankfully rare) cases when babies are battered, it is usually when they cry and parents have not been able to stop the crying. These are usually parents who feel they have no good experience of parenting inside them to draw on.

From parents . . .

Sometimes his crying is so intense that it sets going a vibration in me. My pain gets stirred up by his and I worry that my pain will then amplify his. That's what happened when I was little. When I was feeling pain my mother would feel pain, but it was not an empathic response, it was an automatic reaction. Sometimes she would get angry if I was upset or she would shut off from me, wash up with her back to me, but mostly she would try to "gee-me-up" with an anger-driven hysterical happiness. She would hold on to me and to happiness like her life depended on it. I had to comply. She doesn't do calm happiness. The hardest thing for me is to resist the urge to rush in and quiet the awfulness for my baby. I know that he needs me to hear it and bear it rather than chase it away.

Parents also may feel that they can't comfort their baby if they are on their own, lonely and feeling that someone else should be there to help them. The resentment towards the missing person for not being there can get in the way of dealing with the baby. Single parents can feel like this, as can parents who don't have the support of their own parents. If you feel like this, it is important for you and your baby that you find a friend or professional to help you through this bad patch. You won't be criticised; everyone needs support at times. In fact, people are relieved to get a chance to be involved. It is worrying for outsiders to see a mother and baby suffering but feel that they would be interfering if they tried to help when they're not invited to do so. Most mothers have a worry that people will want to take the baby away. Like feeling guilty when you see a policeman, though it is not rational, it is quite powerful. If you can let people in, you will be reassured that they don't want to take the baby from you but to help you and your baby settle down with each other.

Colic

When a baby's crying seems completely inconsolable, it is often called 'colic.' The crying inexplicably develops into violent and rhythmical screaming attacks. Colic generally begins in very young babies, when they are about two weeks old, and may go in a cycle peaking at two months and usually disappearing by three months, or four months at the latest. When a baby has these screaming attacks, she may scream frantically and relentlessly for two or three hours daily, often at about the same time each day (usually late afternoon or evening). The crying is different from crying at other times of day, with a higher, more intense pitch and with spaces between the cries. The baby may not respond to the usual comforts or respond only temporarily; she stiffens her whole body, arches her back, thrashes her limbs, clenches her fists, draws her knees up to her abdomen, and makes facial grimaces, all of which make her look as though she is in pain.

These screaming attacks can make parents feel panicky. You may feel upset and helpless and can easily become angry. This particular kind of intensive crying really gets into anyone who hears it. You are likely to feel demoralised because you can't calm the baby and criticised or rejected by the baby for not getting it right. The irritated feeling in the baby's body is illustrated by an irritating cry, which makes the parents also feel full of an irritating pain. So as well as having to deal with the baby's state, you have to deal with your own feelings stirred up by the crying so that your response does not exacerbate the problem.

What causes colic?

The baby's body movements often look as though she has wind, and one theory is that it is painful wind caused by an immature digestive system. Another theory is that the baby's pain is the *result* of taking in air during the crying, not the cause of it. The suggestion is that colic is ordinary crying that has got out of hand and then escalated into this desperate kind of crying.

Does it help if a parent thinks of a colicky baby as one having a difficult temperament? It might help move on from feelings of personal failure to the problem-solving of dealing with difficult behaviour. However, there is a danger in thinking of the baby herself as 'difficult' or 'naughty.' An important principle in thinking about human beings is how innate characteristics are affected by our relationships. To some extent, we *all* have difficult temperaments and rely on our family and friends to neutralise some of the more extreme signs of this, and babies need their parents' help in this way. However, babies are not just a reflection of their parents' care; they are also separate individuals with their own strengths and vulnerabilities.

From research . . .

Dr Howard Chiltern (2013), a neonatologist, believes that colic is overwhelm. He does not suggest that parents of babies with colic overstimulate their babies. He argues that some babies struggle more than others with the fact that we are all born 'prematurely' from an evolutionary perspective. Most mammals still go about on all fours, which means they have a nice straight birth canal and their brain size has not increased with evolution in the way that our *Homo sapiens* brains have. This means that they get to stay in the womb until they are ready to be born. Human brains are not fully formed until two years, at which point birth would be impossible. Chiltern argued that the sequela of this prematurity is that we are not born ready to process our physical environment. The womb is full of physical sensations, tastes, sounds, and smell, but there is almost no visual stimulation and very limited social stimulation. Colic tends to start at around four to six weeks, which is when most babies start to get more interested in their environment – looking around, smiling, and engaging people and toys – and by evening they are over stimulated. Not only is this the age that colic tends to kick in but it is usually at its worst in the early evening, after a long period of daylight and arousal. Chiltern also cited the association between colic in infancy and migraines in adulthood as suggestive of both being about sensitivity to overstimulation, perhaps particularly visual and social stimulation. Chiltern argued that the same thing helps – a darkened room, no demands, and a friendly presence! He also pointed out that colic tends to stop at three months, which is when most babies can start to regulate visual stimulation by choosing to look away or zone out. Until your baby has learned to do this, you may need to do it for him. As well as removing stimuli that would not have been present in the womb, it might be helpful to simulate some intrauterine experiences. Many parents intuitively know to rock the baby, as he would have been when mother walked around, to dim lights and even make a rhythmic shushing sound, which simulates the sound of blood being sent around mother's body. Chiltern's advice is to be there but don't try to engage him visually or elicit a to-and-fro interaction. Just be there.

Colic and feeding

It seems that colic is rarely caused by a gastro-enteric problem, so changing the method of feeding is not usually the answer. Breast-feeding mothers do not need to worry that their milk is causing the problem, and bottle-feeding mothers do not need to keep changing the formula.

The upset of the baby crying can make mothers lose confidence in themselves and keep trying something different. Sometimes, if mother and baby have not gotten into a comfortable feeding relationship with each other, this can lead to tentative positions for feeding, where the baby does not latch on effectively. Such feeds could be experienced as 'indigestible.' Taking in wind while feeding at breast or bottle might be a consequence of this uneasiness or awkwardness in the way the baby is sucking. Perhaps an anxious baby gulps too quickly or strains away from the mother's body as she sucks. However, perhaps it has nothing to do with how you and baby come together for a feed. If you are able to keep an open mind to the fact that it might be partly about that, without being hard on yourself or your baby, you might find that you can work your way out of these difficulties.

Mother and baby often need a sympathetic person to help them get together in a comfortable way. Certainly, a mother with a colicky baby needs the father, or someone else, to take turns holding the baby. Often, a father can calm a baby when a mother can't. This need not mean that he is a better parent but rather that he can give the baby a fresh start, away from the tension built up in the previous few hours between baby and mother. If both parents get the same reaction from their baby, there is no escape from the fraughtness, but if one parent can succeed in calming the baby, that can also be upsetting for the other who has 'failed.' It is helpful to think that one parent has to go through the intensity of feeling what the baby has been unable to deal with and the other parent is able to give the baby a respite from this. Being the one to receive and bear the baby's communication of pain is just as heroic, if not more so, than being the one who breaks the cycle.

It may save your sanity to know that colic doesn't go on forever so that you don't let it completely overshadow your relationship. Try to have pleasant interactions with her when she is not crying. It can be tempting to enjoy respite from one another, but you also need to be building up a bank of good experiences together to see you through the tough times.

Should you leave a baby to cry it out?

Some parents worry about responding immediately to their child's crying for fear of 'spoiling' her. Little babies need to be responded to; they don't become spoilt by being picked up and comforted. Confirming your love and reliability is part of the whole relationship that will grow between you and your baby.

It is not that a baby should never be allowed to cry. If a baby cries and is properly attended to, she needn't be picked up again if she cries for a few moments after being put down. As she gets older, she may need some firmness and a chance to soothe herself. Encouraging her to use other comforts such as a thumb or teddy bear can enable her to take charge of her own emotions. This is not a question of leaving her to cry but of allowing her the chance to be separate and to feel and express her mood.

From research on infant crying . . .

Research suggests that responding promptly and appropriately to the crying of very young babies actually reduces the amount they cry later on; it makes them feel more secure and able to explore and confidently enter into other relationships later. What's more, leaving a baby to cry will make her more and more fretful and less likely to respond to your eventual attempts to calm her (Bell & Ainsworth, 1972).

How to calm your baby

Holding

As we have said, holding a baby upright, tightly against your body, often works. Even a baby can sometimes feel psychologically as though she is 'falling apart,' and crying can be an expression of this. Holding a baby physically can help her to feel emotionally 'held.' She may also feel that what she is going through in her body can be felt in the body of the parent holding them. A baby who is kicking and thrashing about all over the place may be relieved by firm holding. There is evidence that desperately crying babies may be over-breathing. If held face to face with a parent, they can breathe in carbon dioxide from their exhaled breath, and this may have a physiologically soothing effect. Alternatively, some parents find themselves holding the baby outwards to get a view of things outside. Looking out of the window may help both parent and baby to get out of a claustrophobic, stressed, shared state of mind. Other babies may not be able to bear too much handling and you might have guessed that your baby is one of these. Maybe you and your baby need some relief from each other. Putting a baby down in a safe place – his cot or pram – and walking a short distance away can give you both a chance to recover.

Dummies

They can work miracles, but not always.

From parents . . .

I can't think why now but I had not liked the idea of giving him a dummy. At two months I tried one out of desperation. It completely resolved our sleeplessness problem. There is no more to say than that.

Someone suggested a dummy might help her to get to sleep off the breast, but every time I tried putting one in her mouth she would make a funny face and spit it out.

I can still remember feeling desperate when one of my babies wouldn't stop crying, deciding to try a dummy and, I must confess, even practically ramming it into his mouth. He calmed down immediately; the fury between us disappeared. I could see how the sucking focused him.

The baby who feels emotionally all over the place is calmed by the neurological process that sucking sets in motion. She gathers herself together through the focus of her sucking mouth. It relaxes the movement of the guts and major muscles while the regular, rhythmic stimulation from the mouth reduces the random thrashing about. Some babies are able to find their thumb or fist; others need a dummy. There doesn't seem to be any good reason for not using a dummy with a baby who needs extra sucking. Sucking has emotional signifi-cance similar to the way the baby is in contact with the mother when at the breast. Sucking on a dummy can represent a memory of sucking at the breast when separate from the mother between feeds.

From parents . . .

At home I don't mind her asking for a feed when she isn't really hungry, it's just like a special cuddle, but in public places it can be quite a hassle getting her latched on in a discreet way. When she then hears something interesting going on and pulls off sharply – leaving me hanging, literally! – I feel really annoyed.

Sometimes I know he's not really hungry; then I think I'm being used as a dummy.

Babies who cry a lot, or who have colic, can often be calmed by sucking on a dummy. The effect can be instantaneous: as the baby starts to suck the thrash-ing about of limbs stops; it seems as though the sucking focuses the baby physiologically and calms him emotionally. Thumb sucking can be equally successful.

Parents may, however, worry about giving their baby a dummy to suck. Does it look as though they haven't been able to satisfy the baby? They may feel 'shame' about dependency feelings and may worry that it will become a habit that will be difficult to break.

From parents . . .

I felt mortified. I was afraid of being made redundant.

Thumb-sucking is fine, it's natural.

I'd rather he had a dummy, at least then I can take it away when the time comes.

A dummy is not a good idea when it is used to shut a baby up; that is, to stop sounds of protest that are a communication to parents. Older babies can be delayed in talking if their parents' reaction to noise is to shove a dummy in their mouth. It stops the exploratory sounds that a baby makes as part of the process of learning to talk. Constant use of dummies can delay the develop-ment of the mouth muscles that are needed for talking.

Teddies and blankets

Teddies are a different kind of comforting object. They come into their own when babies are older and starting to deal with the idea of separation from their parents.

From psychoanalytic theory and clinical practice . . .

Teddies are sometimes thought of as a 'transitional object' (Winnicott, 1958). Transitional objects are one way in which a baby gets through this stage of becoming more separate. A teddy, some other toy, or perhaps a blanket may become special to the baby, particularly at bedtime. It always needs to be there before the baby can settle to sleep. Tiny babies do not have these security objects – they need to have their mother with them for much of the time. These objects come into their own when the baby is in a period of change; they help the baby to start to feel separate while still in close contact with their parents. They do not replace the parents but are a bridge between them.

From parents . . .

I found that giving him my own T-shirt, still smelling of me, seemed to soothe him.

Parents cannot, however, choose which toy or other object is going to be important to their baby; the baby finds its own meaning in something, and this in fact becomes its first 'possession.' As the baby gets older, this possession may need to be carried around, and the whole family recognises its importance.

From psychoanalytic theory and clinical practice . . .

I have noticed that when parents and a baby are having particular trouble in separating, especially at night, parents are often feeling that only *they* can comfort their baby. Although parents can't choose their baby's special possession for them, suggesting that a teddy could be a comforting person-substitute in helping an older baby get to sleep can sometimes allow the parents to see the possibilities. One mother joked with her baby, 'Here's teddy. Give him a cuddle to help him get to sleep.' Her baby seemed to be relieved to be allowed to get on with it and was able to settle.

As with dummies, babies will usually give up their teddy or blanket when they are ready to; they can help a baby eventually to become more independent, not less. Toddlers may use them as an anchor as they go out into the world.

If a child really goes on being rigidly addicted to any of these, she may still be having trouble with separation issues and perhaps the family need to think about the meaning of this. However, many adults still enjoy special objects that anchor us.

Massage

This can be a very comforting, physical way of organising your response to your baby's distress but should not feel intrusive. You need your baby's 'consent' to touch him as much as if he were an adult. Done respectfully, massage is known to improve interactions between carer and baby and to be a protective factor against postnatal depression (Glover, 2001). Perhaps the mutual creating of a rhythm together by mother and baby has a neurological effect that is healing to the mother as well as the baby. The learning about and responding to each other physically enhances each one's emotional state.

Rocking

Rocking is an effective way of stopping rhythmic crying. Gentle, rhythmic motion, about the speed of a very slow walk, helps to calm a baby's heart rate. Perhaps the rhythm first attunes to the rhythm of the baby's crying and then is able to take the baby out of its agitated state of mind and body. Some parents find that an agitated baby can be similarly calmed by being pushed in a buggy or driven in a car. However, they can then find themselves driving around at night to get their baby to sleep and to keep him asleep. This can be very useful short term, but if it continues it may be a desperate measure and a false solution and perhaps represents something about getting out of the house away from the emotions built up inside or of one parent feeling that they need the other one to take the baby away, out of the house. Less extreme, going into another room or out of the house can change your baby's mood and yours. If you tell the baby what you are going to do – 'Come on, we're going for a walk' – you can help her feel that you have some ideas for a fresh start.

Swaddling

Swaddling is an old-fashioned practice that has been rediscovered. It affects the physiological state of the baby and, through this, her emotional state. When babies are wrapped in a tightly folded blanket, they sleep more, have fewer startles and have a lower heart rate variability than nonswaddled babies. This may be effective because the tightly bound cloth recreates the feeling of the wall of the uterus holding the ever-growing baby tighter and tighter during the last period in the womb.

From parents . . .

My first baby was, at the suggestion of the midwife, wrapped in his shawl. A peaceful look came over his face each time he was wrapped up; he would close his eyes and fall asleep instantly. After a few weeks he struggled to have his arms out, though still liking his body to be closely wrapped. As he got older and his movements increased, the shawl soon worked loose and the calming effect lessened but was no longer needed. This did not work at all for his younger brother, who preferred from the beginning to have freer movement of his limbs. This was a very simple example, for me, of how babies' temperaments differ and of how they have their own distinct preferences, right from birth.

Singing

Sounds are important to babies, especially their parents' voices. Babies in the womb can hear their mother's voice and can recognise it soon after birth. Tapes can also be useful to soothe a baby and ones with a heartbeat sound are now available. But parents singing to their baby is the real thing. They can moderate the rhythm and pitch to what they perceive the baby is responding to. The sound is so personal, and the particular melodies and words can have a private meaning between them and the baby. When you sing to a baby, he will often, at the same time, fix you with his gaze, as though he is 'listening' with his eyes. Sometimes parents find that loud music of their own choice will absorb some of their own anger with the baby for making noise, and even though it's not the conventional idea of soothing music it might help everyone calm down.

Bouncing a baby

Sometimes the heightened feelings between parent and baby mean that your 'rocking' gets taken over into a fast, strong rhythm so that you are bouncing or jigging her up and down. If this starts off as getting into tune with the rhythm of her crying, she will feel that you are with her. You will then be able to steady the rhythm, and this may calm her. However, if you find that you are always 'jiggling' her, this may demonstrate the tension inside you and, in turn, make her feel more tense.

If you are ever tempted to shake your baby, put her down safely and walk away. Shaking your baby can cause serious injury.

Carrying

Babies who are carried more in the early months cry and fuss less later on.

Mothers and babies who are close to each other for long periods have a chance to learn about each other and respond. However, mothers who carry their babies also have to work out when the time is right for letting the baby be more separate and start to manage their own feelings.

From research on attachments . . .

One study also found that when babies were carried close to their mother's bodies in the first two months they were more likely to be securely attached emotionally. This made more difference than whether they were breast- or bottle-fed.

From psychoanalytic theory and clinical practice . . .

In her book *Saying No*, child psychotherapist Asha Phillips (1999) described a mother and baby who have had difficulty in letting go of each other. Mother and baby have a good relationship despite a difficult birth, but he hates being put down and 'whimpers as soon as he is out of contact with her.' She ends up carrying him in a sling all day while she does her chores. 'What began as pleasurable contact . . . turns into an inability to part. . . . He seems stuck on to her, even occasionally like a parasite, living off her rather than relating to her. She feels this has nothing to do with who she is, as an individual, and finds him most irritating at times' (Phillips, 1999: 11). By always responding to his whimpering by picking him up, the mother is reinforcing the idea that he can't manage without her. Once a baby has a good bank of experiences of being comforted to draw on, 'saying no' to him can liberate him to discover that he can manage a little independence. He will need this space between them so that they can get to know each other as separate people.

Crying is not criticism of you

Try to remember the following points:

- Your baby is complaining to you, not at you, and her cries are not a criticism of your parenting.
- She believes in you and thinks you can make her feel better.
- She first needs you to know how she feels. This will start to make her feel a bit happier. It gives you time to sort out what she needs.

- It will help her to know that you are getting in tune with her feelings if you can tell her in words what you think she is feeling and what you are trying out to help her. Your tone of voice tells her more than the words.
- Putting it into words helps you to feel that there is some limit to what is going on between you. It is no longer endless misery.
- It might help you to help her if, as you hold her, you try to remember a time when someone listened to you and made you feel better.

There will be many times that you never discover what was the matter, but your job was to bear it with her all the same.

References

Bell, S. H., & Ainsworth, M. D. S. (1972). 'Infant crying and maternal responsiveness'. *Child Development*, 43: 1171–90.

Boutaleb, J. (2019). 'The becoming of a mother. The good enough mother'. [Podcast] *Podtail*. May 3. Available from: https://podtail.com/podcast/the-good-enough-mother/32-the-becoming-of-a-mother [Accessed 06/03/2022].

Chiltern, H. (2013). 'The colicky baby: myths, medicine and making sense'. Available from www.bing.com/videos/search?q=howard+chilton&&view=detail&mid=CE46 C387AE43B50723E6CE46C387AE43B50723E6&rvsmid=ECA7B9EE3F82C9A9 C73AECA7B9EE3F82C9A9CC73A&&FORM=VDQVAP [Accessed 2013].

Fraiberg, S. H., et al. (1980). '"Ghosts in the nursery": A psychoanalytic approach to the problem of impaired infant-mother relationships'. In: S. H. Fraiberg (Ed.), *Clinical Studies in Infant Mental Health, the First Year of Life*. London: Tavistock Publications, p. 417.

Glover, V. (2001). 'Infant massage improves mother-infant interaction for mothers with post-natal depression'. *Journal of Affective Disorders*, 63: 201–7.

Phillips, A. (1999). *Saying No: Why It's Important for You and Your Child*. London: Faber and Faber.

Schore, A. N. (2001). 'Effects of early relational trauma on right brain development, affect regulation, and infant mental health'. *Infant Mental Health Journal, Special Contributions from the Decade of the Brain to Infant Mental Health*, 1–2: 201–69.

Winnicott, D. W. (1958). 'Transitional objects and transitional phenomena'. In: D. W. Winnicott (Ed.), *Through Paediatrics to Psychoanalysis*. London: Tavistock and Hogarth Press.

13 Your baby's emerging sense of self

Originally a chapter from Finding Your Way with Your Baby *(2015), co-written with Alexandra de Rementeria.*

Being a parent is a role that is always changing. From the beginning, babies need to be closely and reliably looked after. This gives them the security to become independent. Then they need the space to develop that independence. This will not be a neat, linear process and there are no general timescales to follow. It is about being in touch with a baby's changing needs. As your baby's capabilities grow, his sense of self also changes. Parents and babies interact differently as the baby becomes mobile and develops a 'mind of his own.' This process, of course, continues through childhood, with adolescence being the real testing ground of whether secure attachments have enabled successful independence.

Temperament and a readiness to relate

'Selfhood' is something that emerges out of interactions with others. However, your baby does not come as a blank slate. Babies are born with their own temperament, which will affect their behaviour, right from the beginning, which in turn will influence the care they receive.

We have seen that babies quickly come to expect you to engage with them conversationally. Newborns imitate tongue poking and a nine-month-old will enjoy teasing you. They are born ready to relate; their interactions quickly become quite sophisticated. Many parents have an intuitive understanding of their baby's capacities and get on with getting to know their baby without giving all of this any conscious thought. If you are feeling a bit flat, it might not come so easily, but it can be motivating, spurring you on to get involved with your baby if you can persuade yourself to notice and believe in his active desire to get to know you.

DOI: 10.4324/b23125-17

From research on temperament . . .

Temperament is thought to be a collection of individual differences that are genetically inherited and manifest as behaviour tendencies from early infancy, and remain stable across different environments and life stages. Temperament is not related to differences in cognitive ability; it is the genetically inherited first building blocks of personality. Personality is the outcome of a complex interaction between temperament and experience. Experience can modify or exaggerate behavioural tendencies, and behavioural tendencies will affect the kinds of experiences a baby will have.

Piontelli (2004) did long-term observations of several sets of twins in utero, using ultrasound scans, and continued to observe them into their third year. She discovered that twins showed distinct temperaments and patterns of relating to one another that were still observable into their third year.

Pregnancy, before separation

In pregnancy the mother's body is performing certain vital functions for the foetus. There are two bodies but they are not yet divisible. Even at the physical level things are not clear-cut and emotionally things are even less clear. It is normal to feel a bit confused about whether the foetus inside you is a part of your body or something separate. However, a mother who has particular difficulty with this may be more afraid and unwilling to face the next stage of separation, which is birth itself. The birth is a 'letting-go' by the mother of the baby into his own individual existence.

Birth as a separation and a coming together

The birth establishes two conflicting truths. The baby is now demonstrably physically separate, but the mother is now much more aware of his dependency on her because she must act to meet his needs, whereas before her body had just got on with it. Some women feel that they have lost themselves, the demands of the baby eclipsing all that formed their previous identity. Some feel that they have lost the baby; others feel that they are getting to meet the baby. You will probably experience all of these feelings at different moments.

Mother and baby as one unit

Babies are born with their own temperament and their own experiences of the womb and of birth but, in many ways, they are not yet their own person.

From psychoanalytic theory and clinical practice . . .

Winnicott (1964), who was so good at memorable phrases, said, 'There is
no such thing as a baby,' adding, 'only a baby and someone.' In previous
chapters, we have looked at the implications of a baby's absolute dependency on adults for survival in terms of how they experience inattention as a
threat to life. Winnicott was interested in how this dependence was experienced in terms of a developing sense of self. He went on to clarify that when
he said that there was no such thing as a baby, he meant that at the beginning
the 'unit is not the individual, the unit is an environment – individual set-up'
and the self emerges from the total set-up, not the individual.

We all have an approximate understanding of this idea that baby and mother
are two parts of one unit because a lone baby just doesn't look right. If in the
street or park you see a baby sitting in a pram, apparently alone, you will most
likely check until you have mentally connected the baby with a watchful adult.
For a moment, you will have been on guard on behalf of that baby, even if the
baby was not doing anything to attract your attention.

You and your baby's emerging sense of self

A newborn is a part of a unit in that he is not yet viable in isolation. He is also
not yet capable of experiencing himself as a 'self' because his brain is not mature
enough; his prefrontal cortex has not been wired together to allow such higher
cognitive function. What of the other half of the unit? You existed before this
new person started to grow inside you. How and why, then, do you become a
part of this new whole? The state of 'maternal preoccupation' described earlier, a
state of powerful identification and obsessive concern with the needs of the baby,
can lead to an experience of merger with the baby. Such a moment of merger
seems to be captured in the following box. The mother found herself bringing
her hungry baby to the breast, despite herself and her wish to follow a routine.

From psychoanalytic observations of babies and parents . . .

Baby cries and mother picks him up. It seems to me that she instinctively
holds him in a feeding position. He starts to mouth. She says that he may
be hungry, but she is reticent. While stating that it is not really time for
his next feed, she brings him to the breast and all three of us relax. He
becomes still and drops off, waking and feeding, and going back to sleep
in a blissful cycle.

The observer went on to explain that when the three 'relaxed,' it was as though a communal hunger had been sated. The baby's wish was felt by the adults, almost as though it had been their own, and the mother's body acted independent of her conscious thoughts and even defying the words she spoke. Perhaps in this moment the baby did not experience his mother as a separate individual to whom he needed to communicate a need, any more than she experienced a conscious decision to meet it. It seems that the mother had lost some autonomy in the service of his needs, almost as though he could bypass her self-will and take up control of her arms to get the feed he needed. An idea mentioned earlier was that the selflessness of parenting is made possible by this identification with the baby. The well of altruistic love is replenished because a part of you feels as though it were your own needs being met. An unconscious fantasy that baby and self are one seems to serve both baby and mother.

From your baby's perspective

We know that a newborn cannot have a mature self-identity, but we can only guess at how he does experience himself and others. There are two different views on whether a newborn feels separate from his mother or not: one view is that he feels 'fused' with her, as though she is an extension of himself and as though her breast that appears when he is hungry really belongs to him. However, the recent research showing that infants recognise their mother by sight, sound and touch straight away suggests awareness, from the beginning, of her as a separate person in her own right. There must be some appreciation of the 'otherness' of the mother to want to bridge the gap by 'talking' to her.

From psychoanalytic observations of babies and parents . . .

This ten-day-old baby looked like he came to feel merged with his mother during a feed. As his mother got him into position to suck, his eyes were wide open and he looked up into her face. While he fed, mother and baby gazed at each other. Gradually, as he became fuller, his limbs relaxed, his eyes lost focus, and by the time the feed finished he was snuggled into her body with his eyes closed.

The infant's body can 'melt' into the mother's body at times of falling asleep, whereas in a more alert state he will be clearer about his mother and himself being separate persons.

From parents...

The second time I left my five-month-old with my mother for a couple of hours he blanked me when I returned. After much singing, coaxing and kissing he finally stopped avoiding my eye and allowed himself to smile. This may seem quite unremarkable except for the fact that the very first thing we had done on my return was to have a breastfeed. I had known he would be hungry and barely noticed myself putting him to the breast before really trying to say hello.

It does seem odd that a baby would be happy to feed from someone he won't look at. Perhaps he did perceive his mother as someone separate, who could disappear and therefore needed to be punished, and yet the breast had a slightly different status, more like something of his that his mother had wandered off with. Perhaps this reflects the fact that the reality is rather paradoxical. The baby is able to recognise separateness at times and at other times lapses into a sensation of merging with mother. Your baby will need you to be open to merge with him at times but also be capable of noticing his attempts to understand your separateness from one another.

Being in touch with your baby's feelings and his self-regulation

To your baby, you will seem to be the whole world at the beginning. Through your attempts to understand what he needs he comes to feel that the world is a place that can know and accept him and his feelings. A parent who is in touch can take in feelings of loving and hating, understand them and help her baby manage them. So, your baby arouses intense and passionate feelings of all kinds. To many mothers, it is all in a day's work to receive them and give back to the baby a sense of understanding and an idea that these feelings can be put into perspective. Repeated instances lead him to remember this and learn how to manage to deal with his feelings on his own. This is the baseline for all relationships in the future and determines whether he will grow up able to temper his emotions or be at the mercy of them.

Being in touch with your baby's feelings and his self-awareness

We discussed elsewhere the significance of imitation, turn-taking, and joking for bonding, language development, and play. These experiences are also crucial to a baby's emerging sense of self. It has been argued that to come to know that we exist, we need to experience existing for others.

To recap, then, being in touch with your baby's feelings enables you to help him manage them now and in the future. It lets him know that he exists for you, which is how he comes to know that he exists in the world. This is part of the higher cognitive function that is made possible by the prefrontal cortex getting wired together. This happens after birth and then only really effectively within good-enough relationships.

Some distance between you can be a good thing

Once your baby has come to trust in the world as a place that is reliably responsive to him, he will be developing a sense of self as reflected back by that world. To develop his sense of self and a sense of agency, he will also need a little space. One kind of thinking about very young babies suggests that they divide everything into 'good' and 'bad' (Klein, 1946). When the mother is there, offering a feed, she is 'good'; if a hungry baby has to wait a while for a feed to come, he may feel that she is 'bad' and leaving him to starve. Gradually, as he has repeated memories that she does always turn up to satisfy him, he will be able to look forward in her absence to the next feed. By 'absent' we are talking about a mother who is actually within reach, perhaps bustling about in the kitchen, stopping the potatoes from burning before dashing to her baby's side! The point is that through these experiences he comes to know that he can have helpful thoughts, that he can be satisfied, for a time, by the *idea* of a mother who will come.

From research on 'readiness to relate' . . .

Trevarthen (2001) showed that newborns have 'intrinsic motives for companionship.' They appear to want to engage with others for the sake of it:

Even a prematurely born infant can, if approached with sufficient gentleness, interact within rhythmic 'protoconversational' patterns in time with the adult's vocalisations, touches, and expressions of face or hands, turn-taking with the evenly spaced and emotionally enhanced movements that are characteristically displayed by an attentive and affectionate adult. They are not only selecting support of internal physiological regulations, nor are they only responsive to caregiving that aims to directly regulate emotional displays (Trevarthen, 2001: 100).

If this getting-into-a-rhythm-together happens even when the baby has no need of external support with how he is feeling, it would seem that the purpose is simply to show the other that you are aware of them and what they are doing. But what bearing does this have on the emergence of self?

Studies of so-called feral children, those found living wild with animals, have shown them to lack certain self-reflexive functions. They don't seem to have an objective sense of their own existence, only their experience of existing so that they don't even recognise themselves in mirrors. It is argued that it is through protoconversations, which can only be had with other people, that such self-awareness develops. Initially, through expression-matching and then mutual imitation, the infant is given the experience of being the object of his carer's attention. 'This experience leads to anticipation, for a contingent and therefore directed-at-me act, and this anticipation is so psychologically and physiologically stimulating as to awaken a new level of consciousness' (Zeedyk, 2006: 329). Reddy (2008) described how we can see evidence of that new level of consciousness as it emerges from such interactions when we see a baby take pleasure in teasing. When an expectation is confounded, in that moment of I-know-that-you-know-that-I-know – something that is not manifest – we know that the joke relies on the presupposition that there is a mind that contains a thought about the content of another mind. Hobson (2002) described this as the 'primordial sharing situation between infant and carer,' from which the infant comes to 'distil out self and other as persons-with-minds' (258).

From psychoanalytic theory and clinical practice . . .

It has been pointed out that there is a logical connection between absence and thought itself. Bion (1962) proposed that tolerable frustration, initially in the form of the absent breast, gives birth to the first thought, in the shape of a wish for the breast. If his hunger is always immediately met, there is no opportunity to have a thought about what is missing, only the experience of hunger followed by feeling sated. However, if the absence is intolerable, then the baby will be too pre-occupied with his frustration to have the thought. A parent needs to allow just the right sort of gap at the right time. Luckily, most will do this without any conscious awareness of how carefully attuned they are to their baby's stage of development and mood in a particular moment.

Language can bridge gaps. One person not knowing what the other is thinking is a spur to use language. A little benign neglect can create the space needed for certain kinds of development. Giving this space is important.

From parents . . .

I use loads of language with my daughter, always describing what we are doing, putting words into context, the physical world, our feelings – everything. As a result, her comprehension has always been amazing, but she is still not talking. I think it's because she knows that I know what she's thinking. She knows she can point and grunt and I'll know just what she means.

Though many mothers find themselves slowly but surely trusting that their baby can manage a little more frustration with time, others struggle to make a judgement. A father can often be the one to suggest that the time might be right. Sometimes the demands of a growing family release a mother from being too attentive in servitude to the baby.

From parents . . .

Looking back it is quite funny to think about how the holy grail of the routine dominated life with the first child, then it becomes completely irrelevant with the second because of all the other demands – toddler's classes etc.

Having never left my first child to cry or settle herself to sleep, when my son was born and needed feeding at her bedtime, she would scream blue murder. I would be in the next room feeding our son and crying my eyes out while my husband tried to comfort her. I thought this was evidence that her heart was breaking when I failed to go to her. I was really worried about how I was going to parent two children. I was then really shocked when, within a week, she was calling for her dad at night, not me.

In fact, absence is a necessary part of any relationship. We talk about getting a look at something from a bit of distance, of 'getting things in perspective,' and babies also need time away from a close relationship to get an emotional perspective on it. Appreciation is sharpened in absence.

Boutaleb (2019), a perinatal psychologist, explained that just as being with the baby triggers brain changes that support the task of mothering a new-born, time away from baby is needed to support the reversal of some of these changes. You will need to be ready to accommodate your baby's need for more independence as she gets older. To do this, you need to hold on to a part of yourself. Your baby will need the part of you that is distinct from her, the part of you that did not become merged with her during bonding. She will need this separate part of you to be available to her so that she learns about herself as separate and how to relate to others as separate people.

Twins and emerging selfhood

This is all so much more complicated when negotiating your relationship with two emerging persons. The mother of twins must balance her desire to treat each child the same, with her wish to allow individuality. This requires not only acknowledging differences in them but also allowing her attention to them to be responsive to their individual needs. It can feel an impossible task to provide an equitable experience whilst fostering individuality. All families with more than one child will face this dilemma, and the difficulty of intense rivalry between siblings for parental attention can lead to a split in the family. The children might take one parent each, as it were, and become possessively identified with that parent. For some parents, a similar defensive split can happen, in their own minds. This allows the parent to experience all of their loving feelings, undiluted by their mixed feelings, in relation to one child. Parents may then begin to feel that their negative feelings have been provoked by the more challenging child, rather than being an ordinary part of all relationships.

Developing a sense of others

In the early months, your baby is still pretty much egocentric. He sees his mother as being there for him. The phrase 'at home alone with the baby' is often used and contains an interesting paradox. A mother with her baby is not alone and yet the baby does not perceive the complexity and richness of who she is in the way an adult partner in an intimate and demanding relationship might, and his personality is still unfolding. In time he does start to perceive her more and more as her own person with feelings of her own, which he might take into account. He starts to see the effects of his actions on her and to have some concern for her. A simple example of this is the one we have described of the baby at the breast who has cut his first teeth. His pleasure in his ability to bite means that he is likely to have a nip at his mother's breast, by accident or not. At this stage, he is able to see that he has hurt her, that other people feel pain, and to be sorry about it or upset if she is angry with him.

Another instance of having other people's needs in mind is the delightful game where a baby of nine months or so 'feeds' his mother or father from the spoon he has just learnt to hold. It is rewarding when your baby does this; it seems like his grateful wish to give something back for having been fed.

From psychoanalytic theory and clinical practice . . .

Creativity may be sparked in the company of others but often needs solitude to flourish. Winnicott has also written about the ability of a baby to be alone in the presence of the parent; that is to be able to play, or follow a train of thought, in the security of the parent's presence but without having to check back at every moment on the parent's knowledge or approval of what he is doing.

How to be alone

One of the main tasks in becoming separate is how to be alone without being lonely. If a parent is always there, the baby may never have the opportunity to be in a room on her own, thinking her own thoughts. Many families don't have the luxury of space but, where possible, sometimes to be on one's own is an important experience.

The connection between physical and emotional development

As your baby begins to sit up unaided, he is literally in a different position in respect to the rest of his family. As a tiny baby he had to be helped to sit up, with his head specially supported. It is an entirely different way to view the world and your family if your own backbone is supporting you and if your head doesn't wobble. Previously, a bouncer chair may have allowed him to sit separately, looking on, but this is not the same as the achievement of sitting up independently. Similarly, when he is placed on the floor, he will be practising turning over, perhaps flexing his knees, and intentionally reaching out for objects.

When a baby is able to crawl, to stand up, and then to walk, life has really changed. Babies need to practise these accomplishments over and over again. It can look obsessive to anyone watching, but this is personal triumph and needs to be done in the context of a relationship. Your delight in seeing your baby start to crawl is part of the joy of the achievement.

As well as attaining motor development, babies in the latter part of the first year are feeding themselves, starting to talk and moving with intention to get what they want. The ways in which they can express themselves are increasing in every direction. All of this changes your baby's feelings about himself and about his relation to others in the family.

Growing independence – leads to doubts

Soon the pleasure of crawling and walking includes moving away from the parent. Independence is at hand. However, a baby who crawls away from his parent needs to know they are there to come back to.

Babies who are practising moving away from their parents need their continued presence to return to. We see this again in adolescence when young people, in the first stages of leaving home, are affronted if their parents are out when they unexpectedly pop back for a visit. In fact, teenagers probably rely on the idea of a parent at home worrying as their protection while they tackle the dangers of the outside world.

From psychoanalytic observation of parents and babies ...

One nine-month-old crawled out of the kitchen into the living room. She turned back and her mother, who had only moved to the other side of

> the kitchen, was out of her sight. The baby wailed dismally until mother called out to her and quickly came back into view.

Independence and adventure bring a backlash of feelings of insecurity, and babies who have always slept well may be more wakeful during this period, sometimes crying out in their sleep as though having bad dreams. They may refuse to let parents out of their sight, and we might guess that their own urge to move has made them worry that their parents are also anxious to escape. Of course, they may be partly right. Once the baby can manage to do more on his own, the tie between him and his mother and father lessens. As they feel he needs them less, they may have thoughts of taking on extra commitments in their own outside lives. Mothers can be surprised to find that although the baby can happily move away from her, he may panic if she moves away from him.

At this point, you will be feeling a bit more separate from your baby, because he is able to start thinking about being separate from you. Paradoxically, he may make more fuss when you go out because he has a better idea that you, as this person separate from him, have left him. However, he is also better able to manage the time apart and to anticipate your return.

At about eight months, your baby may be upset just at the sight of a stranger coming near or even, embarrassingly, a close friend of yours whom he hasn't seen for a bit. This new anxiety does not mean that he has only just started to recognise you and tell the difference between you and other people – he has known you for a long time. It does mean that he has started to realise that you and he aren't stuck permanently together, and he might worry about others getting between you and him. As his mind develops, he has more curiosity and is fascinated by what is new. Through this he has more anxiety as to who and what other people are about. You will often notice that he looks to you to check whether or not to approach the stranger and will be guided by your reaction. He is learning to take clues from you about who is friendly and what is safe.

Giving your child the space to explore

Security and the ability to explore confidently come from being in the presence of attachment figures, the people he is closest to. Your baby needs to know that you are interested in what he is doing and that you approve of it. Babies pick up their parents' anxieties. As your baby starts to move about, to crawl, and walk, he will frequently check with you for feedback on what he is doing. If you give him clear messages about what is safe and what is not, he will learn from this and feel that you are able to protect him from danger. He will then start to get a feeling inside of how to keep himself safe and his own judgement about this will develop. It is important not to confuse him with too many messages that the world is a dangerous place. He needs to learn how to explore safely, not to be stopped from discovering. He will understand from your tone of voice and expression that it is dangerous to touch certain objects, such as electric sockets; if you use these vetoes sparingly, he will usually respect them. However, as a baby becomes mobile, it is necessary for parents to simplify their home and make it as safe as is feasible. He needs to be shown how to climb safely on furniture, not to be stopped from doing it. Always saying 'no' to a baby can crush their spirit of exploration.

It can feel as though your baby is no longer under your control – always on the move, making a noise or a mess, starting to be defiant, closing their lips if they don't like the food offered, waking up at night when previously they've been good sleepers, getting into everything or getting at them. A docile, grateful little baby has become her own person. This stage may be a delight, but it can also be a big shock for parents. Parents who have felt themselves to be beautifully in tune with their baby can feel very 'out of sync' now. Increasing independence sometimes coincides with the end of the weaning phase, with mothers and babies losing their special relationship with each other. A mother may feel that the baby is now part of the wider world, not just belonging to her, and both parents may have to grapple with the realisation that their baby now has a mind of his own. Exploring together with a parent is also important. Going out and coming back home differentiates 'home' from 'outside world' and reinforces an idea of self in relation to the place and people he belongs to.

From parents . . .

When we come back from our walk he looks up at the window of our flat. He knows it's his home.

Conscience

Babies at the end of the first year start to have a moral sense, a feeling of what is right and wrong, in relation to their parents. This moral sense goes along with the development of the baby's capacity for self-reflection. He gets to recognise his own states of mind through his parents' interest in them. He then progresses to realising that 'there are other minds out there' and he, in turn, can perceive his parents' states of mind. He starts to realise the effect that you and he have on each other. It matters to him that you approve of him, and he will regulate his behaviour accordingly. Babies do have to experiment, both with what it feels like to do something and also what your reaction will be. If your baby throws some food on the floor at the end of his meal, he is working out cause and effect on different levels: the laws of gravity and the rules of parents! You have the difficult task of working out the balance of encouraging self-expression and deciding when enough is enough.

This negotiation is the basis for many future workings-out of the balance between freedom and compliance. One major arena in the following year will be the beginnings of toilet training. Success in this is a toddler's achievement of self-regulation and wanting to please his parents. It need not be a matter of 'discipline.' It is a mistake to try to toilet train a baby in their first year; they are too young to understand and give consent to the process. The time to toilet train is when a toddler can recognise his own bodily signs and has his own words or signals for needing to do a 'wee' or 'poo,' because the control of bodily functions is matched by control over language.

Gender and identity

We have spoken about the importance of the fluidity of roles and functions in a family; the idea that it needn't be the father or even a man who complements the mother's role is familiar. Yet there is a biological necessity for an actual male, or at least his sperm, at conception. The idea of a parent of each gender seems to persist in the minds of children, even when all of their needs are being met by a single-sex family. Perhaps this has something to do with needing to know oneself in relation to each gender, in an intimate way, in order to know who one is, to have a fully rounded sense of self.

From lesbian parents . . .

We are a lesbian couple and we adopted my partner's niece when she was taken into care due to her parents' drug and alcohol problems. She knows she has a tummy mummy and a daddy who we don't see because they're not well, then us – her two forever-mummies. My partner and I both noticed her watching a little girl playing with her daddy in the park and we felt it was important to acknowledge her interest in them. She has asked if she will see her own daddy when she's big. She is very curious about her uncle and has a really special bond with her grandfather.

Another lesbian couple had a baby through sperm donation, and the process of choosing a donor raised interesting questions about the formation of identity. They had agreed that given the limited information offered on sperm donors, his age was probably most important because of improved chances of healthy sperm. Yet, they were both drawn towards an older donor who had said a few words about his motivation for donating sperm. They came to realise that they had not only his sperm in mind but an actual person who their unborn child might seek to make contact with at age 18. They were confident that between them they could provide what their baby needed but they could still keep a space in mind for a child's wish to know his or her biological father. The business of genetic inheritance and how it affects emerging identity is also an issue when choosing a donor.

From lesbian parents . . .

My partner had never wanted to carry or give birth, but I guess I was conscious of her not getting to pass on her genes because I found myself wanting a donor with her colouring. She seemed totally uninterested in this at the time, but I do think it is hard for her now when we see that our baby is starting to look like my mum, for example.

When family members note shared genetic characteristics, it is a sort of claiming that might underpin a baby's emerging sense of himself as belonging. However, these things are rarely straightforward. The mum quoted earlier was reassured to remember that another lesbian couple they know found that their baby looked like her biological mum but grew up to have her other mum's character. After all, identification is an ongoing process, much more complex and fluid than a simple looking-like the other and often has more to do with the roles taken up in the family.

From lesbian parents . . .

My partner feels a much stronger impulse to thank our donor and more curiosity about his features and about whether our son has siblings through him. It is hard to know whether that is because he represents her contribution – the other half of the genes that aren't mine – or whether it is because I'm the stay-at-home, breastfeeding mum that she then identifies with him as "the father," the one in the other role.

References

Bion, W. R. (1962). *Learning From Experience*. Lanham, MD: Rowman and Littlefield Publishers.

Boutaleb, J. (2019). 'The becoming of a mother. The good enough mother'. [Podcast] *Podtail*. May 3. Available from: https://podtail.com/podcast/the-good-enough-mother/32-the-becoming-of-a-mother [Accessed 06/03/2022].

Hobson, P. (2002). *The Cradle of Thought*. Oxford: Macmillan.

Klein, M. (1946). 'Notes on some schizoid mechanisms'. In: *Envy and Gratitude and Other Works 1946–1963*. London: Hogarth Press and the Institute of Psychoanalysis (published 1975).

Piontelli, A. (2004). *Twins, From Foetus to Child*. London and New York: Routledge.

Reddy, V. (2008). *How Infants Know Minds*. London: Harvard University Press.

Trevarthen, C. (2001). 'Intrinsic motives for companionship in understanding: Their origin, development, and significance for infant mental health'. *Infant Mental Health Journal, Special Contributions from the Decade of the Brain to Infant Mental Health*, 1–2: 95–131.

Winnicott, D. W. (1947). Reprinted in Winnicott (1964) *The Child, the Family and the Outside World*. London: Pelican.

Zeedyk, M. S. (2006). 'From intersubjectivity to subjectivity: The transformative roles of imitation and intimacy'. *Infant and Child Development*, 15 (3): 321–44.

Part 5

Reflections

14 Enlivened or burnt out

Originally given as a paper at the Paris WAIMH Congress in July 2006.

Every mental health institution has its own version of the old joke 'How do you tell the difference between the patients and the therapists? The patients are the ones who get better!' I am going to argue the contradiction in this. Perhaps the therapists are the ones who stay well by working with their patients.

Let us first look at what we mean by burn-out. Kennerley describes 'burn-out' as an anxiety disorder. He says, 'This term describes a reaction to chronic stress, which is particularly common among caring professionals' (Freuden-berger, 1974). This stress can be 'positive' such as overwork, pressured deadlines, or impossible targets, or 'negative' such as job boredom, lack of autonomy, or frustration. Symptoms are similar to the other anxiety disorders but tend to be more marked because the stress is ignored or dismissed until it has reached a debilitating level. It may be ignored through habit or because stress is construed as 'excitement' or because an individual's drive over-rides their awareness of stress. We don't have to go far to recognise this!

Monica Lanyado (1993) has pointed out how vulnerable we are to stress and distress in dealing with raw emotional experience. She says that the

> work is often felt to be a vocation and is therefore deeply rooted in the strengths and vulnerabilities of the individual's personality. In this respect many of the most dedicated workers would find it impossible to think of any other kind of work that could be more satisfying.

It is interesting to note what our daydreams are of what we might otherwise do. Are we planning to run a restaurant, idealising our creativity and unlimited resources, but still at the beck and call of endless hungry customers, or do we prefer to fantasise that we have the quick wits and guiltless greed to survive in the world of high finance? Lanyado quotes Alice Miller to show that those of

DOI: 10.4324/b23125-19

us in this work might be especially 'gifted' in being sensitive to the difficulties of our parents. Are we doomed to go on understanding them, or trying to understand our own predicament, through empathy with others? Or conversely projecting our problems into these others?

Working with infants and their families must have a profound effect on us workers. We may feel the pleasure of helping inter-generationally distressed families manage a 'fresh start,' or we may feel dragged down or fragmented by the repeated communication of disturbance and distress.

A formal psychotherapy training and personal analysis may help workers recognise where their own vulnerability may be triggered by that of patients. Primary care workers without a specific mental health training need supervision and support. Working in a baby clinic, I see how life and death feelings are part of the ordinary state of the clinic. Parents who have had a baby are normally in a heightened state of being. Professionals have to stand the anxiety of this, and evaluate when some of this is out of the ordinary and needs special attention. My consultation to doctors and health visitors includes helping them to tolerate the stress without rushing in to action, or conversely I may help raise the anxiety level where necessary. Avoiding taking on emotions may lead to burn-out.

Working with postnatally depressed mothers requires a particular state of mind in health visitors and others. Some of these mothers perplex the worker, irritate, or anger them. They may make them feel they have 'got it wrong.' Consultation gives the health visitor a chance to discover that this may connect with the mother's experience of not being understood by her own mother. Feeling understood, the mother may be able to understand her baby better; the worker also feels less dismissed and useless. However, a health visitor brave enough to listen to a postnatally depressed mother will hear shocking material, such as hatred towards self, baby, or partner, and fears of damage. Support for the worker is needed here.

In most psychodynamic kinds of work, it is taken for granted that our own experience is stirred up by the work with patients. Oddly, however, this has not yet totally permeated the wider early-years professions. In AIMH-UK, we have succeeded in being part of the advisory committees for government departments, producing, for example, training materials for all workers with children. These documents do now acknowledge the importance of the relationship between worker and child. But they only describe the effect of the worker on the child (except in work with abuse). We Infant Mental Health professionals add in to the drafts of the documents the effect of the child on the worker. Again it is left out. This seems to be a difficult concept. Our view that thinking about mutual interaction makes it more manageable has not caught on at the top bureaucratic level. Some people in management have risen from the ranks of workers and have kept a spirit of generosity towards those still at the 'coal-face' – their caring now is for the professionals. Others, perhaps burnt-out themselves, are defended against tangling with emotion and want to keep to 'targets' and closely defined tasks, and resist opening 'Pandora's Box.'

However, many of us teach professionals who seem relieved and inspired to take on thinking about the personal effect of their clients or patients on themselves.

Research in CAMHS (Child and Adolescent Mental Health Services) on the Therapeutic Alliance looks promising (Green, 2006). It shows that this alliance is reliably measurable and (modestly) affects treatment outcomes. It quotes Carl Rogers back in the 1950s suggesting that the emotional quality of the therapeutic relationship was the main agent of therapeutic change within psychotherapy and includes the patient's experience of 'accurate empathy.' Recent work on task-related alliances such as in CBT includes the patient's appraisal of the therapist's credibility, enthusiasm, and commitment. This research is really useful, but it does not tell us the effect of the therapeutic alliance on the therapist.

I would like to return to the opening joke. I suggest that the therapist can actually gain from therapeutic alliances over time with many different patients and develop personally, while being able to start again at the beginning each time. Picasso said, 'If you know exactly what you are going to do what is the point of doing it?' I believe that as therapists, however experienced we are, seeing patients keeps us vulnerable. Every patient changes us a little. Margery Brierley said that the aim of analysis is to let the patient make the discoveries. But alongside the patient, we also make discoveries. Freud pointed out the use of humour in psychoanalysis, and other writers cite wit and surprise. Both parties need to be genuinely surprised. As in Stern's description of attunement between parent and infant, something new to both must come out of an encounter – each party has lived a little and has changed each other.

What do we specifically get from our work in infant mental health? In parent-infant psychotherapy, we often have the pleasure of attuning to viable families. Ed Tronick (1989) talks about the 'normal, often occurring, mis-coordinated interactive state as an interactive error, and the transition from this mis-coordinated state to a coordinated state as an interactive repair' (p. 116). Tronick is talking about interactions between parents and baby. I think this also holds true between therapist and the families who are our patients, and that the repair may be as therapeutic for us as for the patients.

As well as attuning to families at ease with their infants, we must also stand not being in tune with parents who are treating their babies badly and not condone their behaviour even while understanding how it comes about. Attunement to the child in such cases may have its dangers for the therapist. Beebe (2002) has noted that when mothers demonstrate non-attuned behaviour (such as intrusiveness), their baby's heart rate goes up. As therapists, our blood pressure may be affected as a matter of course by getting in the way of these misdirected attunements! Kalin et al. (1995) have shown that in primates, attachment behaviours operate on the brain of the mother as well as on the brain of the baby. How intimate need the contact be to have an effect? Perhaps even in a professional situation therapist's brains are at risk from other people's disorganised attachments!

However, more optimistically, Regina Pally (2000) argues that 'it is known that consciously attending to and verbalising something can enhance cortical functioning, and take advantage of its plasticity, to modulate deeply engrained emotional responses' (p. 15). Pally is writing about intensive psychoanalysis, but I suggest that in parent-infant psychotherapy where we touch, albeit briefly, on deep early processes, major psychic changes can also occur. I suspect that there must be equally an emotionally integrative effect for the therapist who goes through such a process with parents and their infants that is deeply satisfying.

References

Beebe, B., & Lachmann, F. M. (2002). *Infant Research and Adult Treatment: Co-Constructing Interactions*. London: The Analytic Press/Taylor & Francis Group.

Freudenberger, H. (1974). 'Staff burnout'. *Journal of Social Issues*, 30: 159–65.

Green, J. (2006). 'Annotation: The therapeutic alliance – a significant but neglected variable in child mental health treatment studies'. *Journal of Child Psychology and Psychiatry*, 47: 425–35.

Kalin, N. H., Shelton, S. E., & Lynn, D. E. (1995). 'Opiate systems in mother and infant primates coordinate intimate contact during reunion'. *Psychoneuroendocrinology*, 20: 735–42.

Lanyado, M. (1993). 'Stress – an occupational hazard of working with disturbed children'. *Educational Therapy and Therapeutic Teaching*, 1(2): 23–38.

Pally, R. (2000). *The Mind-Brain Relationship*. London: Karnac Books.

Tronick, E. Z. (1989). 'Emotions and emotional communication in infants'. *American Psychologist*, 44: 112–19.

15 Saying what you mean, or meaning what you say

Originally published in the Association for Child Psychotherapists' **The Bulletin.**

As Alice in Wonderland declared, 'That's the same thing you know.'

I sometimes wonder what the articles in the Bulletin really mean. There seems to be a lack of genuine critical faculty in some of the accounts of papers read at our own meetings or other conferences. Is it really appropriate to describe our 'delight' or 'gratitude' at hearing these 'excellent papers'? What about some good-mannered intellectual appraisal?

Gabriella Klein had the unenviable task of reporting on my own paper on feeding problems at the 1996 Annual Conference, after hearing me expostulate on sycophantic write-ups. Gabriella has done a very decent job of giving a clear description of my main arguments with no superlatives. She also included the discussant Tessa Baradon and ideas from the floor as part of the occasion. She then gives some new thoughts of her own, developing ideas in the paper. Struggling now to rewrite the paper for publication, I am grateful for her useful summary but could have done with some thoughts on its deficiencies! But my point is that with obsequiousness out of the way Gabriella's creativity could emerge. I do think that this is a serious issue and that our profession is prone to self-infantilisation both within its ranks and in relation to other disciplines. When the ACP was founded in 1949, it was greatly helped by John Bowlby, who made a case to sceptical medical colleagues for this equivocal new profession. However, the cost was the self-deprecating title Association of Child Psychotherapists (non-medical). I was on the Executive when, in March 1972, in what seemed a daring act of liberation, we dropped the 'non-medical.'

I don't count myself as immune from the process. When Mary Boston and I produced a draft of our book 'The Child Psychotherapist,' Dieter Pevsner, the publisher, pointed out that the first word in the manuscript was 'although.' 'You'll never change the world with "although",' he said. One of the best interpretations I've ever had!

DOI: 10.4324/b23125-20

The (self) infantilisation within the profession seems to take place in the teaching system. It is of course one of the essential values of learning, to idealise the knowledge, and thence the teachers who hold it. But our trainees also bring knowledge into the system. Each year I see new trainees arrive as experienced professionals with unique specialised skills but collapse into anxious psychoanalytic novices. It is indeed necessary to abandon defences of 'knowing' already, in order to have the deep satisfaction of learning something new, but I think there may be a culture in all the trainings of playing a game that the tutors 'know' and the trainees don't. When a game like this is played, what happens to truth? Is the younger generation saying what it means, or only what it thinks that its seniors want to hear? Worse than that, do they think we are too fragile for an argument of equals?

Two of the creative geniuses of our work, Melanie Klein and Anna Freud, were notable for their belligerence in their prime, but in old age both were faithfully looked after by friends and followers as though theory and practice must not be challenged. Stephen Mitchell says that Freud himself often constructively changed his own mind, developing new theories, but could not tolerate correction and argument by his younger colleagues, and this seems to have continued in the psychoanalytic system.

On a slightly different note, as child psychotherapists we are likely to identify with the child and perhaps suffer powerlessness from that, and it can become a habit. When we set up the Child Psychotherapy Trust, Susanna Cheal, as its consultant, pointed out how reactive we child psychotherapists always were – we went into a room and waited for someone else to start!

In an old story of my father's, a distinguished Rabbi was visiting the Rabbi of a small town, and found him carefully arranged, washing the feet of a beggar. The Senior Rabbi sat in silence and waited. Unable to contain himself at the lack of reaction the local Rabbi burst out, 'Well, what do you think of my humility?'

Perhaps, genuine or not, humility is an over-rated virtue!

DILYS DAWS

16 Working at the edge

The quiet subversiveness of psychoanalytic thinking

Originally given as a paper at the Capetown WAIMH Congress in June 2012.

Einstein apparently said, 'Make things as simple as possible, but no simpler.'

Psychoanalysis at its best is about simplicity, and Bollas and Sundelson have a wonderful phrase, 'psychoanalytic quiet.' There may literally be quiet in a psychoanalytic session, or even in a parent-infant psychotherapy meeting with parents, an infant, a toddler, and more than one worker. To pass on this style of working, I often co-work. One health visitor was impressed by how much a depressed mother told us about her difficulties with her children, and about her own abusive experiences. The health visitor, however, confessed, 'At first I couldn't stand the silences!' I thought 'What silences?' I had been occupied thinking about what the mother told us. When a patient tells you something important, you may need to be silent so that they can also think, and so that they can say the next thing on their minds. Free Association needs another listening mind.

In a busy parent-infant session, we may all find ourselves silently watching the baby. And in this shared moment some key emotion about the problems is revealed.

Genius is about making complexity simple. Daniel Stern connected psychoanalysis and child development. The idea of affect attunement is about expressions or behaviours that show we understand the emotions of the other. In playing with a baby, we match our movements to his, perhaps imitating, perhaps translating into a different mode, and then spontaneously we move on to a new set of actions that capture the spirit of our engagement but take us somewhere new. We may do something discordant, Stern's purposeful misattunement. Then it gets boring, we look away, and take the feeling of mutuality into different activities, or indeed to being separate.

DOI: 10.4324/b23125-21

We need to look at where attunement stops working. A postnatally depressed mother may miss some of the signals from her baby and be preoccupied with her own feelings – or she may be able to attune well to a small responsive baby. The trouble may come when the baby becomes mobile, crawls, and walks away from her. She may feel rejected as he explores the world; she may feel that his lively discovering is out of sync with her own inward-looking mood. As he roams the kitchen, she may feel not only that he 'gets into everything' but that he is 'getting at' her. When he climbs, instead of showing him how to do it safely she may tell him to stop doing it. These are the children, usually boys, who get diagnosed with ADHD, and who have accidents because they do not have a parent's voice inside them, keeping them safe. Discovery and creativity are cut short.

In this work, we go into each family ready to discover what is there. We discover something about the patients and keep ourselves vulnerable. If we are able to attune to the patients, to be with them, we are then ready to create change with them.

Caroline Lindsey, a family therapist at the Tavistock Clinic, talked about curiosity. If you are with the patients, you want to know about them. If you are lucky, parents may then start to want to know more about their babies. Thinking that had become stuck opens up. Do they sense that we are there for all the family? Do they sense that this means that we subversively disagree with their formulation that the baby is the problem and that we are sticking up for the baby as well as for them?

If you are attuning to patients you are attuning to a vast complexity. In working with sleep problems, for instance, I am assailed by a vast array of jumbled emotions, of repetitions of experiences that have not been reflected on. As I have discussed elsewhere, even in brief work allowing your unconscious to be in touch with the patient's, and to receive these feelings, can perhaps help to integrate them. I have compared this process to the integrating process that dreams may achieve.

You are now going to hear about my granddaughter. Noa aged five came to visit in a sulky mood and at first did not speak to me. After a few minutes, she thawed a bit and I asked her to do a drawing for me. She got the materials and rather furiously, but with some humour, applied herself. Instead of the usual flowers and princesses, she drew lines, using every one of the coloured pencils and felt-tips. Someone grumpily said, 'She's wasting ink.' Noa's father said, 'We don't say Jackson Pollock wasted paint!' I said, 'Perhaps Jackson Pollock was making a point to his grandma.' The criss-crossing of lines, the discordance, were perhaps a representation of the cross feelings between Noa and myself, successfully integrated in a very simple picture.

Noa was very pleased with her picture and stuck it on the wall of the sitting room for all to see.

So are subversive and creative the same thing? Subversive means positively turning things over, uprooting. The more negative undermining is only one facet of its meaning.

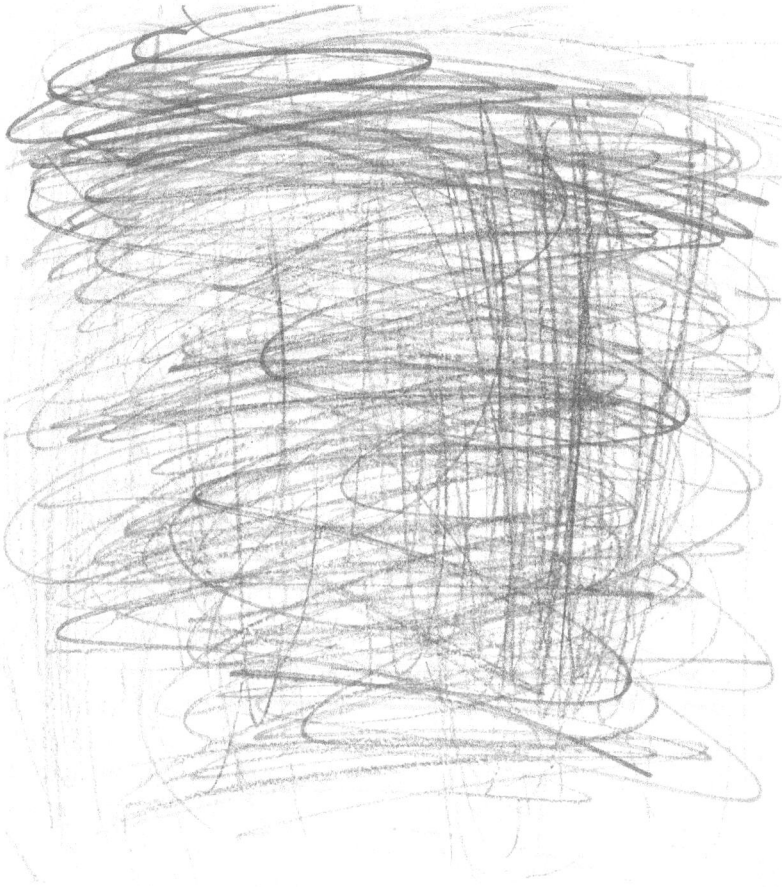

Figure 1.1 A picture drawn by my granddaughter Noa (the original is in colour).

Parent-infant psychotherapy is fairly new, born of the respectable parents of psychoanalysis and family therapy. Was it Stern who said that new populations of patients bring out new ways of working? In work with infants, we are playful, we take risks, and perhaps we compete with each other in innovative practice? Perhaps in brief work with people on the edge, unable to contain their own crises, often suffering disjunction from their original families and cultures, do we take on the outsider status and attack the establishment ostensibly on their behalf?

We need babies to keep the population going, to pass on our genes. We need them not to be clones of ourselves. We even need adolescents to challenge the status quo or we would all atrophy. So do we also identify with the challenges that infants bring, and become subversive in the grown-up institutional world?

Can I go back to my granddaughter's picture to talk about the value of discordance? The US composer Charles Ives's father wrote music for two different orchestras, playing two discordant tunes against each other. It sounds wonderful. Ives took on this discordant theme in his own music. Discordance is an important element in music. It can feel unsatisfactory if it is missing.

Working in the public sector, in the baby clinic of a general medical practice I have often thought that one of the benefits is the access to people who would have difficulty coming anywhere but their own family doctor's surgery. I see very troubled distressed people who are unlikely to change much. But they do get something important from coming to see a therapist. I find myself very drawn to these quirky people and get a lot personally from having to contend with their disturbances, albeit in this protected role. I can get to know about thought processes and emotions that are not, at first sight anyway, part of my own repertoire.

Does one pass on something of this in being subversive in political work?

A crucial way of looking at this is through fairness and justice. Eric Rayner, my husband, has written about fairness and justice in psychoanalysis. Over a short period, he noted the opening themes of his analytic patients and was struck by how many began with a personal issue about fairness and justice. He realised they could have been complying with what their analyst tended to pick up.

In work in the public sector, our patients are even more likely to be the victim of personal or social injustice, and certainly to perceive themselves as being so. Sometimes, we help them to manage it better. Sometimes, we even help patients survive bad housing better.

Do we then get filled with projections and need to pass these on, or do we in fact have evidence of social need and the case for equality and social justice?

In the UK, we have been very successful in political action, in making the government aware of need and in creating innovative Infant Mental Health provision. An NHS that belongs to us all is part of the inspiration for this. Disgracefully, public services are under threat from the current government. We will need all our optimism to reinvent what is being cut and to get back the feeling of equality.

17 Error and repair

Originally given as a paper at the Leipzig WAIMH Congress in June 2010.

This symposium is about what we later realised we had failed to notice in work with patients, or had got wrong. I am also going to look at what felt wrong at the time, or what patients told me I had got wrong, but became part of the theme of the work. But first, what we got wrong in the past.

For my generation of therapists, there is the shame that when we started, we simply did not know about child sexual abuse. We may have worked intensively with some children, who, as the treatment continued, did not seem to get better. They went on being restless, uncommunicative, at odds with the therapeutic relationship, or showing explicit sexual behaviour. Were they psychotic, we wondered? We spent hours in their company but the sad truth is that we did not ask them the most important questions that would have helped them to tell their unbearable, unthinkable story.

One of the patients, Josie, I felt fondest of was an eight-year-old girl in care whom I saw at our Day Unit twice weekly, and then once weekly at the clinic for two to three years. The clinic had close contact with several children's homes in the area. The staff of the home seemed warm, caring, and supportive of the therapy. Josie made a 'home' in my therapy room: on the inside of the door to her locker, she stuck a list of her toys. Twenty years later, Josie, now with two children both on the child protection register, sued the local authority for thousands of pounds of compensation for sexual abuse in the children's home. The case went on for months, years, and nothing was proved. The local authority managed to lose the clinic file with my unsuspecting notes.

Was this a case of abuse, accurately recalled when she had vulnerable children herself, was it opportunistic for the money, or was it a more general feeling that there should be compensation for a childhood spent in care? This wild child was felt to be unfosterable and unadoptable. If there was abuse was it current in the children's home, or earlier in her family? Her escort to therapy loved

DOI: 10.4324/b23125-22

her, and so did I, but only for an hour a week. She was the one child that I had a serious fantasy of taking home and looking after properly. Perhaps I knew that I was failing in what she really needed, understanding and knowledge of her actual experiences.

Now to error and repair, Tronick (1989) talks about 'the normal, often occurring miscoordinated interactive state as an interactive error, and the transition from this miscoordinated state to a coordinated state as an interactive repair' (p. 116). He is writing about interactions between parents and infants, but it may equally hold good in the therapist's attempts to interact with patients.

When patients feel that they have been misunderstood they may well be right, but these perceptions may be an intrinsic part of the work. The feeling of being at odds with each other may have a dynamic meaning. So getting it wrong may be part of the process of getting it right. How comforting that even our mistakes may turn out for the best!

In work at a baby clinic with one mother Jessica and her four-month-old baby Thomas, my faults were soon obvious. Thomas had been born by IVF from an implanted donor egg and Jessica told me of the distress about it not being her baby genetically.

In the first meeting, I collected them from the baby clinic. Jessica was holding Thomas outwards in a sling, and both looked at me. I noticed but did not remark on their likeness. In the meeting, Jessica started by telling me of the implanted donor egg and her distress about this. I said, a bit confused, that I had thought how alike they were, and she agreed that people said that. I asked if Thomas looks like his father and she said he did. I asked if she looked like the father and she again said yes. We had a moment of wondering together about this likeness.

The next meeting was six weeks later after both our summer holidays. Jessica talked more about her feelings about Thomas not being 'her' baby genetically and about Thomas's liveliness, which was apparent and very attractive. I then made my big mistake and said that it was a generalisation but sometimes when mothers were depressed, their babies were very lively to help cheer them up. I immediately felt I shouldn't have said it. A theoretical point, not a timely felt one, and certainly not one discovered between us. The next week they were late. In the room, Jessica said she was angry with me for last time – what I had said about depression and liveliness. I said that I had worried that she wasn't coming because of that. She said, 'I thought you would.' We laughed a bit, but she said she was upset that I was wrong. I said perhaps it was useful that she could think I was wrong but could still come and make use of it. She was then able to talk more about the IVF. She had her baby just before she was 46. She had her own embryos but had had a miscarriage. The doctor said she had a better chance of carrying an implanted embryo to full term. Her own frozen embryos still exist. She also talked about her very difficult critical mother, and I wondered if the decision to use an implanted egg was also to disconnect from her own mother. I had just seen the film *I've Loved You So Long*, where a mother adopts for this reason.

The next time she said how helpful this had been and told me how traumatic the birth had been. She had needed a caesarean, had a haemorrhage, and a blood transfusion. After all this she couldn't move and they said, 'Don't you want to hold your baby?' She couldn't move to pick him up and no one offered to put him in her arms. She said she couldn't bear to look at the birth pictures because she and the baby are apart. They were being looked after separately. I said, 'They were saving your life.' In a later session, she told me her partner was desperate for them to have another baby. I asked if that would be dangerous for her. She said, 'Thank you for asking that.'

My acknowledgement of how life threatening the birth was helped the work become less emergency focused, and we moved on to the separateness between Thomas and herself, and to going back to work in a creative profession that she loves. The conflict between her wish to keep him close, his growing independence, and indeed her own wish to separate brought back some of her agonising about whether he really was her baby. She talked about her fear of having to tell him one day and what that would do to their relationship. I said keeping him so close now was because of her fear of losing him. I said he was supposed to grow up and leave her one day. I said I wondered if it was easier that he wasn't a girl and that carrying a female embryo that wasn't her own might have been harder. Perhaps as a boy he might care less about whose egg it was – that was women's business. She laughed and said her partner thought that too.

There was also a long-haul journey to see the father's parents. She began one meeting by saying how angry she was with me for the previous session when she had told me of her mother-in-law's wish for them to go straight to stay with them. I had no idea what it was like to travel overnight with a baby, be exhausted, and need to recover. I said I had sided with the grandparents, and we both smiled, complicitly.

Why have I chosen this case as one to apologise for? This was a successful, indeed enjoyable piece of work although based on a mother's extreme distress that natural conception could not produce a live baby.

I think that my crass mistake in the second session, of making a probably correct but completely mistimed interpretation was my defence against the distress she had come to tell me about. Perhaps also I had come up with a bit of theory to make up for my profound ignorance of the complexity of IVF. I hadn't previously taken in the meaning of egg donation, and that there are no inherited genes. Jessica's anguish included the feeling that her mother-in-law was blood-related to her baby, while she was not. A colleague pointed out to me that serum passes from mother to baby through the placenta. How much had she indeed made him her own in the womb?

The fact that I could apologise and settle down to attune with her was perhaps helpful in changing her perception of her mother. As I became a therapist who could be wrong but still useful, so her mother changed into someone who offered welcome help and insights. To balance this her mother-in-law became more infuriating. I think the separateness that my mistakes implied also allowed us to look at the separateness between her and Thomas in a less fraught way. When I said, 'They were saving your life' about the birth, she could give up some of her projected fury with the obstetric staff for treating Thomas and herself separately. She could move on to the ordinary life process of separating.

However, I recently saw a mother Mildred and her two-month-old baby Fraser, where I did badly miss the point. Mildred is from a war-torn country. In the UK she has been raped by more than one 'uncle' and has HIV. The conception of the baby was not from a rape and did not cause the HIV. In our first meeting, she told me a story, not of rape but of having been defrauded of all her savings, and being further tricked into getting into debt. Listening to this story of a tragedy unfolding, my blood ran cold. I was physically affected by hearing the story and could hardly bear to listen. It actually felt as bad as many of the stories one hears of rape, or near-death births. I asked about other times when she had been helplessly drawn into a sacrifice of her self and learnt of emotional abuse and denial of her identity. I learnt that the father of the baby had refused to allow the name she had chosen for her son and insisted on one that had no meaning for her. As we talked, I noticed that Mildred rarely looked at the baby. His buggy was placed so that I could not see him and because of the urgency of her story, and the shame with which she told it I did not, as I usually would, pay attention to him.

In the next couple of meetings, she talked of her shame about losing her savings. Fraser's buggy was second-hand. She had lost the money that would have bought him a new one and had to pay back her debts. I was full of indignation on her behalf and told her of the government scheme to help people in debt, including condoning some debts to banks. The health centre had someone who could advise her on this. I see myself as a very sensible therapist in touch with the environment. Mildred said she preferred to pay off the debt.

In a later meeting, Fraser cried and she picked him up and held him to look out of the window. This time I did comment that she did not look at him. She was surprised and said that she had a cold and she didn't want him to see her looking like that. I said she was important to him, and I thought he would really like her to look at him. It did not occur to me to say that she might feel that the HIV has damaged her so much that she doesn't want him to see that. Because of the drugs for the HIV, she is unable to breastfeed him – where has the outrage about this gone?

As Fraser has learnt to sit up, I have asked Mildred to let him out of the buggy to sit on the floor near us both. I played with him, handing toys to him, and taking them back. I invited Mildred to join in and she said how much she enjoyed it. The next time she spontaneously put him on the floor. Fraser looked at me and held out his arms. I said to Mildred that he remembered our game after a two weeks gap.

The shame of the loss of the money seemed to recede and Mildred talked about her return to work. She has a degree and has worked in an admin job, but in the recession seems unable to get back into this. She works as a carer and travels for up to two hours to do piecemeal jobs of half-an-hour to two hours, travelling between clients' homes. I have said how exploited she is letting herself be, and she has started to feel this, and now refuses the half-hour jobs.

Until writing this, I had not noticed how systematically I have avoided talking about the effect of the HIV on Mildred's relationship with Fraser. HIV is an exquisitely shameful state, and is often kept a secret. Patients ask for it not to be in their notes. A GP told me that patients treated in a specialist unit may not tell their own doctor about it. With good referrals, I sometimes feel that I am supposed to know about the HIV but not to discuss it. The loss of a future that the loss of the money represented to Mildred must be much more located in the loss of a healthy body that could nurture her child, and she might always feel she would be a source of contamination and danger to her child.

In the first case I said too much. With Mildred and Fraser, I have not yet said enough. In Bowlby's words do I feel that I am 'Knowing what you are not supposed to know?' How do you talk about what the patient cannot?

Perhaps the message is that self-scrutiny need not spoil the enjoyment of this work but give the patient an example of creatively going on thinking.

Reference

Tronick, E. Z. (1989). 'Emotions and emotional communication in infants'. *American Psychologist*, 44: 112–19.

18 Rivalry with fathers

Originally given as a paper at the Prague WAIMH Congress in June 2016.

In parent-infant psychotherapy we may work with two parents and their baby, perhaps an older toddler as well; often we find ourselves seeing just a mother and baby. There are many reasons for this; father is at work, mother needs time to talk by herself, or she says, 'He doesn't like talking about the problems.' But why are we sometimes secretly relieved to work just with the mother-baby duo?

In this symposium, we look at the complexities of triangular communication (Fivaz-Despeursinge & Philip, 2014), the competition between therapists and fathers as to who understands the mother and baby best, and of where the transferences lie. In fact, so much more can happen when fathers are present in the room.

Over 30 years ago, the psychoanalyst David Malan referred a patient of his to me for help with her sleepless baby. I met with the family and in the first meeting the father who had also been in analysis asked, 'How does the transference work here?' A good question. I am still working on the answer. The baby slept through the night after a couple of sessions, but how we got there was complex. These parents were from different countries, different religions; they had both had difficult life experiences but they were really committed to each other and determined to make life good for their baby. The beginning of each session became a routine. The mother who suffered from postnatal depression would burst into tears saying she was a bad mother. The father and I would then, patronisingly, assure her that she was a good mother, doing the best for her baby. After a couple of weeks of this ritual the mother said, 'Why don't you two go off and get married?' A very timely warning to me not to 'capture' either party of the parents and to remain an outsider for them to use me as they needed to.

DOI: 10.4324/b23125-23

The Oedipus complex is one of the key discoveries of psychoanalysis, the one taken up most enthusiastically into common language. Ron Britton (1991) has described how 'the closure of the Oedipal triangle by the recognition of the link joining the parents provides a limiting boundary for the internal world.' He calls this a triangular space. If the link between the parents – perceived in love and hate – can be tolerated in the child's mind, it allows a third position where the child is a witness, not a participant. If he can observe he can also envisage being observed.

Elisabeth Fivaz-Despeursinge (2008) has pointed out that when babies interact with one parent while having the other in mind, in parenthesis, their minds will become structured for complex thought. You could say that differences of opinion, though not hostility, between parents are essential for babies to experience them as separate people. Just like the baby, the therapist may have to tolerate being a witness, not a participant, as the family endeavours to understand and repair the ruptures in their relationships.

Are Oedipal conflicts in the family thus mirrored in the therapist? Just as the toddler who climbs into the parent's bed feels that if he literally kicks his father out of it he will have the perfect union with his mother, do we, male and female therapists alike feel that we can offer a special relationship to the mother that is interrupted by the father's presence, that he takes away our place. Do we feel that we can manage the mother's views about her baby, but not take on the conflicting views of her partner? We often talk about who is the patient, the mother, the baby, or is it the relationship? So much more complex to manage. Taking on the father as well means that we ourselves are indeed able to see the world in 3D.

When I hear a passionate story of an enmeshed mother and baby, I think of the mother's relationship to her own mother, of possible unbearable separations, and of intense ambivalence of love and hate. But I also wonder about the father's role and why the 'intercourse' between the parents is not sufficiently protective to allow mother and baby to pull satisfactorily apart. There are often mentions of 'male insensitivity.' Progress may be when the marital issues are eased and the mother feels able to take the father's advice.

When mothers come with their babies claiming that father is not interested, does not want to come, I may feel that she is unfairly representing difficulties in the relationship in a one-sided way. In one instance, I urged the mother to persuade the father to come. To my surprise, he was charming, attentive to the mother and baby, and talked cooperatively with me. After this meeting, the mother never came again. Had I called her bluff – that the father was not as she had described? Or had I been conned, and taken in by false compliance? In either case perhaps she could no longer trust me.

In a case that I and my trainee are seeing now, the mother comes with the baby. Both are delightful. The mother loves the baby but is unsure of herself in her maternal role and pines for her exciting work-life. She envies father still able to go out to work, and too busy to come to the therapy sessions.

I suggested, as I usually do, that she tells him what we talk about when he gets home. She says that she worries that she overloads him already with her doubts about herself and her mothering. She comes to see us in order to spare him. Fathers who do not attend can indeed support the mother's work in the therapy but this may be mainly at a conscious level. Having the father actually in the room allows him to work at an unconscious level and, as with the mother, I think working in the presence of the baby is also crucial for the emotional depth of the work.

I have been fortunate to work for a lifetime in the NHS in the UK. I think of the State as a kind of father, helping with authority, setting out boundaries. Working with families who are mistreating their children, it is essential to empathise with the difficult experiences that have led to their behaviour but not to collude with cruel treatment. Without absolving oneself from responsibility, it can be helpful to have this authority in the background. Even with well-functioning families, working in the public services gives a framework of triangular functioning, with the therapy echoing families that include a father.

References

Britton, R. (1991). 'The missing link: Parental sexuality in the Oedipus complex'. In: J. Steiner (Ed.), *The Oedipus Complex Today*. London: Karnac Books, pp. 86–7.

Fivaz-Despeursinge, E. (2008). 'Infants in triangular communication in "two for one" versus "two against one" family triangles'. *Infant Mental Health Journal*, 29 (3): 189–202.

Fivaz-Despeursinge, E., & Philip, D. E. (2014). *The Baby and the Couple*. London & New York: Routledge.

A day in the life of . . . Dilys Daws

Originally published in the Association for Child Psychotherapists' **The Bulletin.**

1. Describe your job/role in one sentence

I retired from the Tavistock seven years ago and feel very lucky to have a profession that enables one to carry on working. I have a portfolio of freelance teaching, consultation, work at a baby clinic, committee work, and campaigning. Most of this is connected with Infant Mental Health. I was the founding Chair of the Association for Infant Mental Health (AIMH), and this area is still my central interest. The greatest pleasure of retirement from a senior post is being able to do just the enjoyable bits, not having administration, and being responsible only for your own work, not other people's!

2. Tell us about a typical day in your working life

Every day is different. One day I teach on the Infant Mental Health Course at the Tavistock. On the days at home, I do supervisions of child psychotherapy trainees from various trainings, some by telephone, consultations for senior therapists running Infant Mental Health Services round the country, and am an advisor to AIMH and on various 'advisory' groups on Infant Mental Health and primary care. One morning I work at the baby clinic of the James Wigg Practice doing parent-infant therapy, and consulting to staff. I love the contact with parents and babies struggling to make sense of their difficulties and this also gives me the live experience and the right to speak on behalf of them, and of the professionals in primary care. I am glad still to be working, with its sociability and challenges. I do less writing, but am still campaigning – I have always thought my family was relieved that my reforming zeal had an outlet outside of home! It is also really enjoyable to have free time, to spend with my

DOI: 10.4324/b23125-24

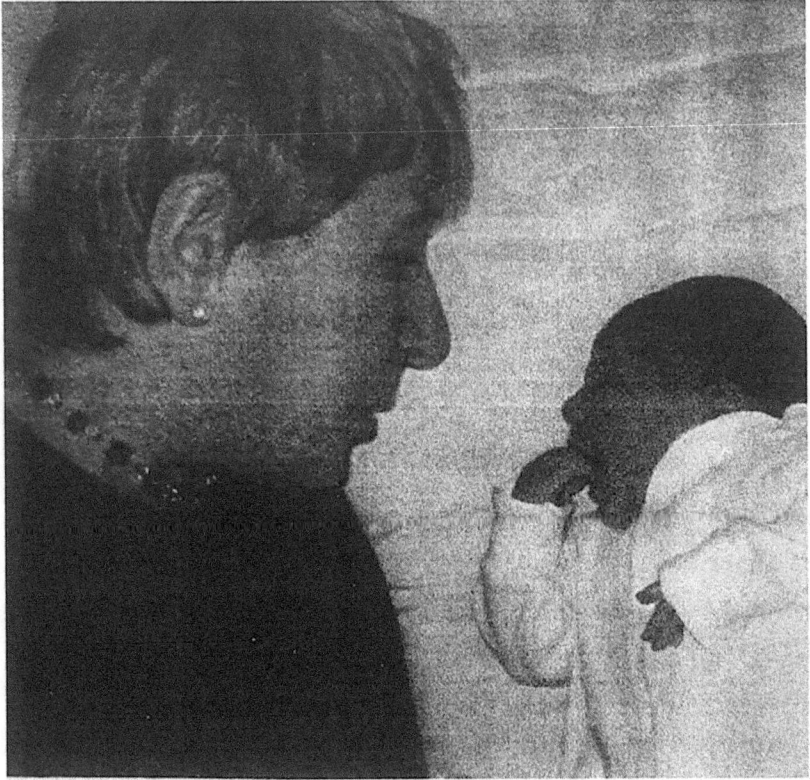

Figure 1.2 Dilys Daws with her granddaughter, Noa.

husband who calls himself a 'happy old man,' with my grandchildren, and time just to potter without doing anything useful!

3. Name three qualities about the geographical area/ location where you live and/or work.

I live in Hampstead, near the Heath, an easy walk to the Tavistock, and am lucky never to have had the stress of commuting. I moved to Hampstead 50 years ago, when I first came to London. I knew the centre from occasional theatre visits with my parents but had not been anywhere else. I was fascinated by what I had read of the artistic, bohemian aspects of Chelsea and Hampstead, but Chelsea sounded too 'posh' for me – so I chose Hampstead and lived in bedsitters. Even when we came to buy a house, it really wasn't expensive in those days.

4. What would you say are the greatest challenges facing you in your area/role today?

Working freelance means needing to keep a coherent framework, not taking on too many diverse tasks, and working with colleagues and teams where possible. I have Honorary Consultant Child Psychotherapist status at the Tavistock and feel backed by them when going out and about, making quite difficult adversarial points at meetings, for example, at the Department for Children and Family Services (DCFS). My peer supervision group also helps to keep all the bits together. Email can be persecuting, but often I find it companionable – Members of the AIMH Committee and Advisers seem to be sitting at their computers at the same time some evenings, and a lot of useful conversation goes on. Being used as an 'elder' also requires being careful not to confuse one's knowledge and experience with a wish to keep things as they used to be.

5. What would you say is the biggest challenge facing child psychotherapists in today's changing political landscape?

I am a natural optimist, and get very confused by what seems like the destruction of child psychotherapy in many parts of the country, when there is so much more knowledge of its value. On the Child Psychotherapy Trust, we worked to make child psychotherapy better known to politicians and the public, and we thus prepared the ground for the ACP to get regional training posts created. It felt at the time that success could only continue and that NHS Managers and families had only to hear about child psychotherapy to be convinced of its usefulness. It seems to me that the public as a whole is much more open to thinking about emotional issues, and particularly children's distress. I may be naïve, but I am hoping that the rise in CBT might lead to its practitioners seeking more training to work more psychodynamically. We nearly all of us came to child psychotherapy discovering the need for it from previous professions and wanting to get to the essence of things.

I am glad that the ACP is once again going on a national campaign about the value of our work. I am personally now involved in a similar situation in health visiting, where the universal health visiting service is under threat. I think the two go hand-in-hand and believe that health visiting is essential to underpin any infant mental health provision.

6. Name one piece of psychoanalytic literature or one psychoanalytic writer that you have found particularly helpful or inspiring.

I can't choose just one. Reading bits of Freud, and Susan Isaac's, descriptions of children at the Malting House school in the university library inspired me to train as a child psychotherapist. Daniel Stern is the writer I now quote most to students for understanding how child development research illuminates psychoanalytic thinking.

7. 'If you knew then what you know now,' what would you have liked to have been different in your training?

I loved my training, but it was narrowly based compared to now. It was very small: Juliet Hopkins and I trained together; a third person became ill and dropped out. We qualified in 1963, the training only took three years, including infant observation. It felt too short and we both stayed on another year, finishing our training cases, continuing supervision, and analysis and going to some of the lectures again. We were taught by the 'greats,' including Dr Bowlby, and having infant observation with Mrs Bick. She used my baby, 'James,' in her paper, I must say without either asking or telling me. I only discovered it when I read the paper in the Journal. Publishing ethics were different then!

Juliet and I trained very young; we qualified before we were 30. It meant that life was less complicated, we could concentrate on the training, but we brought less to it than many of today's more mature students.

What would I change? My idea at the last annual conference that instead of five times a week psychoanalysis, four times a week psychotherapy, and once a week physiotherapy (or Pilates, or yoga) would help us learn more about ourselves has already aroused interest. I only recently came to this myself. When I started Pilates, the teacher said, 'You're all mind, and no body.'

My biggest plea would be for the trainings not to be tempted to infantilise trainees, who sometimes lose some of the experience and authority they had in their previous professions. I know that we all have to lose our arrogance in order to learn, but I think our current difficulty in making an impact on the mental health world could be helped by empowering students more, so that they regain their seniority quicker when they qualify.

8. Do you have a favourite novel or poem you could recommend?

'In Reference to her Children' is a beautiful poem by Anne Bradstreet written in 1656. Miranda Passey showed it to me when I was writing about the issues of being apart from their young children for working mothers. The poem is about a mother bird's relationship to her children, her difficulties about separation, and her working through these. It brings tears to my eyes whenever I quote it in public.

> 'If birds could weep, then would my tears
> Let others know what are my fears
> Lest this my brood some harm should catch

And be surpris'd for want of watch

Great was my pain when I you bred,
Great was my care, when I you fed.
Long did I keep you soft and warm
And with my wings kept off all harm.'

She describes the process of coming to terms with their leaving, and of her own death, and the poem ends:

'When each of you shall in your nest
Among your young ones take your rest,
In chirping languages oft them tell
You had a Dame that lov'd you well,

That did what could be done for young
And nurst you up till you were strong
And 'fore she once would let you fly
She shew'd you joy and misery,

Taught what was good, and what was ill,
What would save life, and what would kill.
Thus gone, amongst you I may live,
And dead, yet speak and counsel give.

Farewell, my birds, farewell, adieu,
I happy am, if well with you.'

On a lighter note, I am also rediscovering irony in reading *The Gruffalo*, or *Not Now Bernard* to my grandchildren.

9. Have you ever thought of changing your profession and if so – what would you do?

Like many of us, I fantasised about running a restaurant, until I noticed that a feeling of pure hatred came over me when my children asked, 'What's for dinner?' There is no easy way to cater for infantile needs. Similarly, I often thought that selling beautiful modern furniture would be a simpler kind of life, until again I realised that people trying to improve their lives with 'retail therapy' might be in very complex internal states, or life situations, but interpretations would not be appropriate! I did think of being a politician, but some years ago I heard Shirley Williams talking about a political defeat, and saying 'I didn't cry.' I wouldn't have made a politician because I would have cried too often.

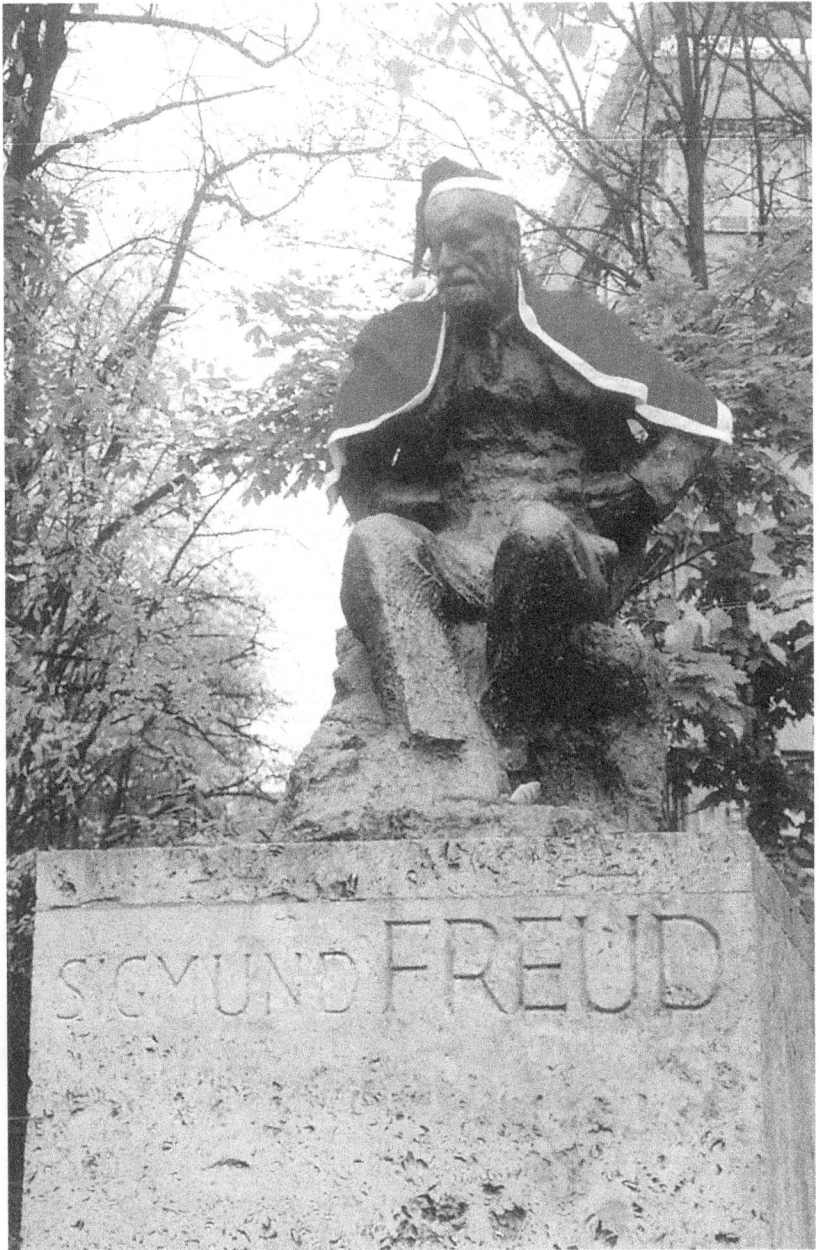

Figure 1.3 A Christmas card created by Dilys Daws, Will Daws & Eric Rayner.

Source: Photograph taken outside the Tavistock & Portman Clinic.

10. If you could choose a character part in a play, who would it be and why?

Cordelia. A couple of other people have chosen her recently. I have always thought I was like her – taking the high moral ground but saying it a bit wrong, being completely misunderstood, and not having the common sense to correct it. I have just been to King Lear at the RSC and had to endure the agony of seeing it all go wrong again.

Historically I have fancied myself as a nineteenth-century reformer, but I expect in reality I would have been caught up in the social constraints of the time, and been glad just to fit in.

Index

For Product Safety Concerns and Information please contact our EU
representative GPSR@taylorandfrancis.com
Taylor & Francis Verlag GmbH, Kaufingerstraße 24, 80331 München, Germany